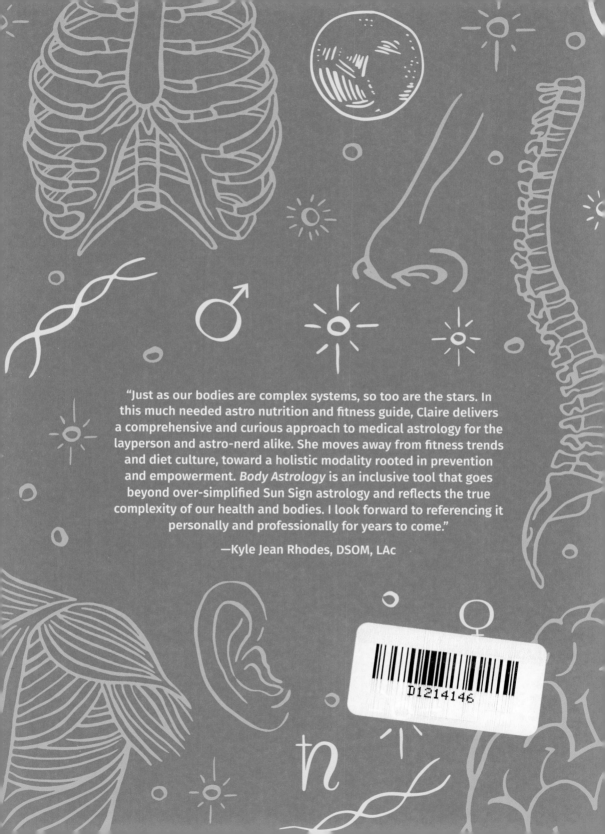

"Just as our bodies are complex systems, so too are the stars. In this much needed astro nutrition and fitness guide, Claire delivers a comprehensive and curious approach to medical astrology for the layperson and astro-nerd alike. She moves away from fitness trends and diet culture, toward a holistic modality rooted in prevention and empowerment. *Body Astrology* is an inclusive tool that goes beyond over-simplified Sun Sign astrology and reflects the true complexity of our health and bodies. I look forward to referencing it personally and professionally for years to come."

—Kyle Jean Rhodes, DSOM, LAc

D1214146

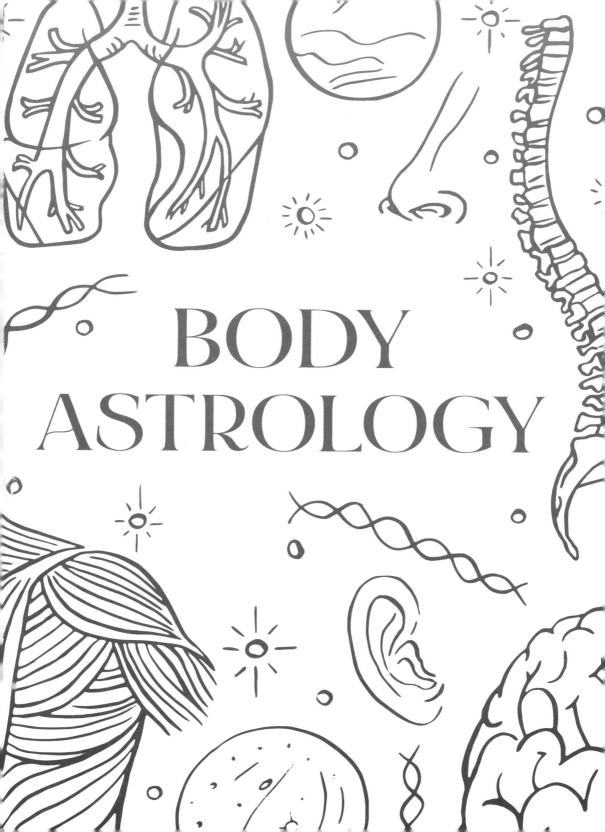

BODY ASTROLOGY

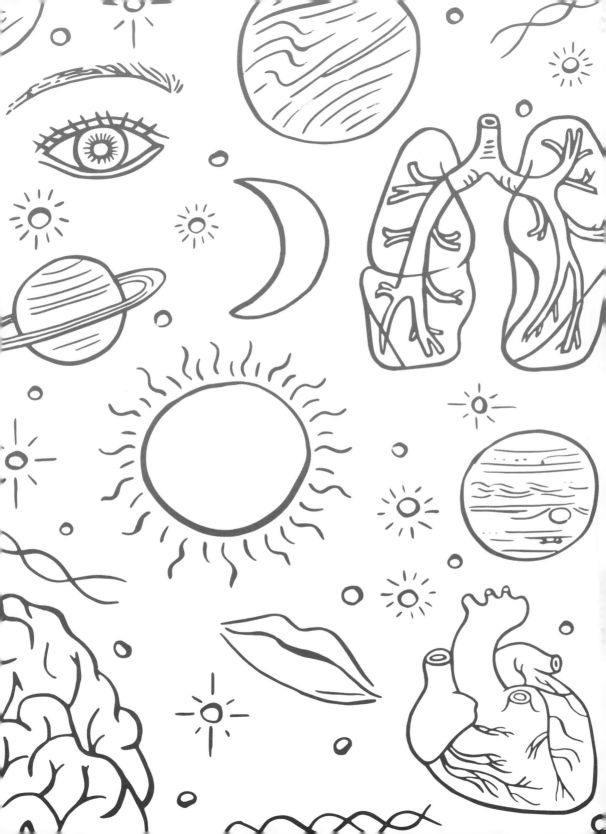

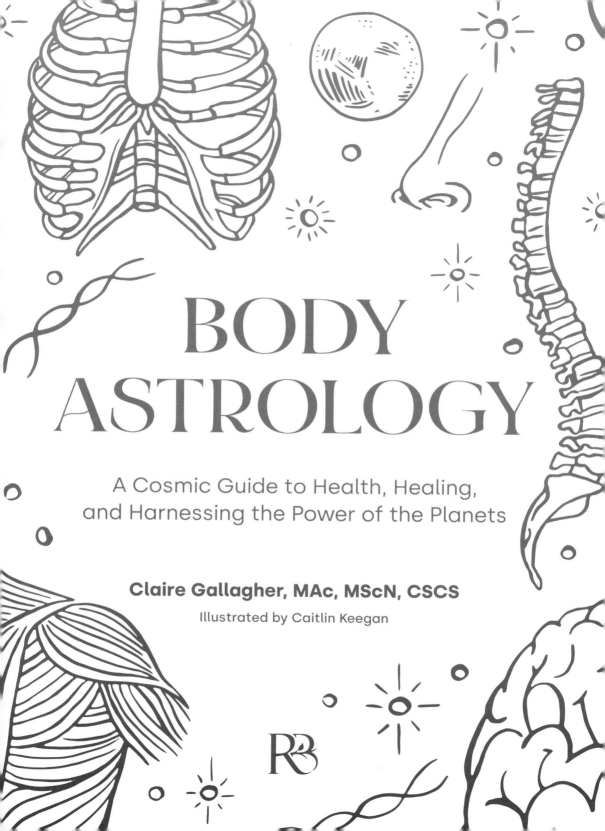

BODY
ASTROLOGY

A Cosmic Guide to Health, Healing, and Harnessing the Power of the Planets

Claire Gallagher, MAc, MScN, CSCS

Illustrated by Caitlin Keegan

RB

Roost Books
An imprint of Shambhala Publications, Inc.
2129 13th Street
Boulder, Colorado 80302
www.shambhala.com

Cover art: Caitlin Keegan
Interior and cover design: Amy Sly

The information presented in this book is thorough and accurate to the best of our knowledge, but it is intended for educational purposes only, not to diagnose or treat medical conditions. Please consult a qualified health practitioner regarding any specific health concerns, movement routines, and personal care. Shambhala Publications and the author disclaim any and all liability in connection to the use of the instructions and practices in this book.

9 8 7 6 5 4 3 2

Printed in China

⊗This edition is printed on acid-free paper that meets the American National Standards Institute Z39.48 Standard.
♻Shambhala Publications makes every effort to print on postconsumer recycled paper. Roost Books is distributed worldwide by Penguin Random House, Inc., and its subsidiaries.

Library of Congress Cataloging-in-Publication Data
Names: Gallagher, Claire, author. | Keegan, Caitlin, illustrator.
Title: Body astrology: a cosmic guide to health, healing, and harnessing the power of the planets / Claire Gallagher, MAc, MScN, CSCS; illustrated by Caitlin Keegan.
Description: First edition. | Boulder: Shambhala, 2022. | Includes bibliographical references and index.
Identifiers: LCCN 2020053713 | ISBN 9781611808421 (trade paperback)
Subjects: LCSH: Astrology and health.
Classification: LCC BF1729.H9 G35 2022 | DDC 133.5/861—dc23
LC record available at https://lccn.loc.gov/2020053713

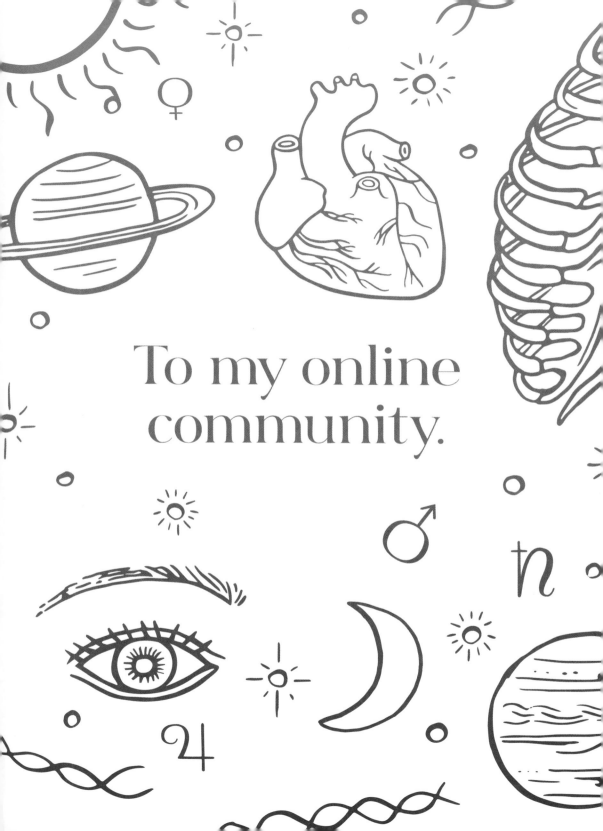

To my online
community.

Contents

PART THREE

The Planets

Introduction

True story—I grew up terrified of astrology. Part of this was the spiritual environment I was raised in, but I like to think another part of this was my budding inner wisdom. I'd go through great pains to make sure my teenybop magazine didn't accidentally fall open to the horoscopes in the back. When it inevitably did, I'd be horrified. Am I really this prudish, uptight, goody-two-shoes Virgo you speak of? That isn't a cool way to be described when you're in seventh grade, and so my hatred for my Sun sign began. I didn't know it back then, but on my birthday, the Moon was hanging out in Aquarius (in astro-speak, we call this your Moon sign). Knowing this, it makes sense why horoscopes were offensive to me. They felt like a loss of freedom, which is one of the quickest ways to infuriate an Aquarian.

My point in sharing my somewhat misplaced childhood fear is that it's totally normal to not resonate with your Sun sign. It's totally normal to maybe even dislike your Sun sign, as I used to. (For the record, I'm now a very proud Virgo.) And it's also totally normal to love your Sun sign but feel that something's missing. That's because something, or *a lot* of somethings, is missing. What many of us are actually averse to isn't a single zodiac sign but the incompleteness of Sun sign astrology.

My astrology fear was healed by illness. In my early twenties I developed a mystery condition that I carried for years. Doctor after doctor couldn't put me in a clear diagnostic box and so I fell through the conventional medicine cracks. I vividly remember crawling through the house on my belly when I was just twenty-one because I was too weak to walk. I was forced to quit my job and move back in with my parents, and I spent much of my time in bed crying. As the years progressed, every organ system slowly developed dysfunction and my symptom list grew unbelievably long and complex.

Like many people with similar stories, this experience led me to the world of alternative medicine. Being sick and without many resources forced me to research remedies and experiment on myself. Like a typical Virgo, I mostly dabbled in nutrition. I made a lot of mistakes along the way, even stumbled into a few dietary fads, but it was undeniable that my most significant improvements always came through food. In fact, repairing my relationship with food got me well enough to where I could start moving again. When I was strong enough, I became a yoga teacher and eventually a personal trainer. Yoga allowed me to enjoy movement while I was still healing. Later, weightlifting fortified my body and gave my delicate nervous system a more rooted home.

Eventually I gathered enough strength to upgrade my piecemeal self-healing experiment and study nutrition professionally. I moved across the country to attend the National College of Natural Medicine with the intention of becoming a naturopathic physician. But while I was there, I fell in love with the elemental language of Chinese Medicine and its ability to articulate my "undiagnosable" experience. I soon found myself enrolled in a dual master's program, studying both acupuncture and nutrition.

One day, rushing between class, clinic, and my part-time personal training gig, I saw in the school bathroom a flier for a medical astrology conference. It wasn't exceptionally flashy, but for some reason it captivated me. Up until that moment, my fear of astrology still eclipsed any interest in the subject. I still thought astrology was about telling the future or putting people in limiting personality boxes. But medical astrology? The physicality of that felt safe to explore. At this point, I had spent four years immersed in Chinese Medicine theory and practice. Associating organ systems and imbalances with elements, seasons, and constellations was an ancient practice that I trusted. Surely Western astrology, although a different elemental tradition, couldn't be much different? Chinese Medicine had softened me up for this fateful bathroom moment. Plus, my lingering symptoms selfishly piqued my curiosity.

I'm sure you can guess the rest. I went to the conference and that was that. Within five minutes of listening to the keynote speaker, who later became my tutor, I knew medical astrology was my thing. As odd as it sounds, I felt like I already knew this system and was suddenly remembering it. In medical astrology, the birth chart becomes a map of your unique body workings, needs, strengths, and susceptibilities. This is invaluable because two people may suffer with the same condition, but because of the differences in their birth charts and bodies, their symptom pictures, emotional experiences, and pathways to healing will differ. I already knew there was no one-size-fits-all in healing, but medical astrology took the idea of bio-individual treatment to amazing new heights.

Medical astrology also deepened my understanding of body rhythm and taught me how to use the planets as healing clocks. As the sky changes and interacts with your chart in new ways, your physical needs and experience change too. This was especially interesting to me as someone who had chronic fatigue, which is often characterized by a monotonous wall of exhaustion and pain, or symptoms that come and go without warning. The chart gave me insight into what was ready to heal, what needed more time,

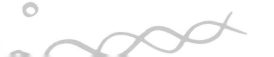

what emotional patterns were involved, and when flares were likely to occur. When you're chronically ill, this information is gold because it allows you to practically and mentally prepare and save your precious energy for what's ripe to respond.

After the conference, I immediately shifted everything to serve my medical astrology study. I kept a nauseating number of planetary symptom journals, gathered the birth chart of every patient who'd let me, started designing movement systems based on the lunar cycle, and enrolled in astrology classes. I was obsessed—because astrology gave me hope. It perforated the narrative that I loved to cling to—that I would always be sick. Did I want to be sick? No. But it had become familiar and therefore oddly comfortable. Astrology gave me the perspective shift I needed to finally open to the possibility of healing. It helped me unearth not only the physical roots of my condition but also the deeper psychospiritual roots. Astrology also helped me navigate the overwhelming world of health care. I finally had something to help me discern which course of treatment might be worth my time and which was just another path to a pile of soul-crushing medical bills.

My medical astrology obsession was then continuously fanned by its creepy accuracy. Hit a personal record in the gym—a Moon-Saturn trine was supporting hard work and strength. Patient comes in with a rash—Mars on the Ascendant, which meant they were more susceptible to acute and itchy conditions. It didn't take long before I could predict my own and others' cycles of health, and my work as a professional medical astrologer began.

I've got to admit—it was a hard sell. The first few years, I felt like a total goofball, yelling into the online abyss about working out with the Moon cycle and supplementing for your Saturn return. If you didn't grow up in an astrology bubble (I sure didn't), you can probably imagine the looks I received. Even in alternative medicine circles it was very fringe and not something people were actively talking about. Building trust with my then small online community became my number one task. I believed that if people could just experience astrology in their own bodies, they'd be on board. So, instead of trying to convince people, I spent my time creating an astro-movement system, sharing my own experiences, and teaching people how to keep astrological symptom journals. Turns out, my hunch was right. As people began observing and *feeling* astrology, they realized how practical it was, and their curiosity exploded. My business grew slowly but organically, and at the perfect pace for this introvert.

Fast-forward some years and I've had the honor of sitting with hundreds of people, observing firsthand how medical astrology provides hope, new perspectives, aha moments, root-cause clues, and healing momentum. But my favorite, by far, is watching relief wash over a person's face as they realize their chart simply gives them permission to be exactly as they are. Astrology inherently challenges the societal definition of "health." We're told that health looks and feels a certain way, while astrology leaves room for the infinite diversity of bodies and experiences. One very small example—astrology challenges the assumption that being "healthy" means you always feel energetic. That's a lot of pressure to put on yourself. Astrology reminds us that the body is not static but cyclical. There are times when the sky is busy (what modern culture often labels as "well") and times when it's quiet. These are both expressions of health.

I don't believe astrology tells you anything you don't already know—although it may feel like that at times. Rather, I see it as an affirming and uncovering tool. It reacquaints us with parts of our hearts and bodies that we may have hidden or forgotten. You can play the game of telling your health future if you want. But the real magic of medical astrology is in its whisper to open all the doors of your body's house and fully inhabit it. When we lovingly look at all our pieces (which the chart is so good at showing us) and give them the attention and nourishment they need, we become our own medicine. Whether you're still on the astrological fence or a total fan, my prayer is that the information in this book leads you to a well of deeper and deeper self-trust.

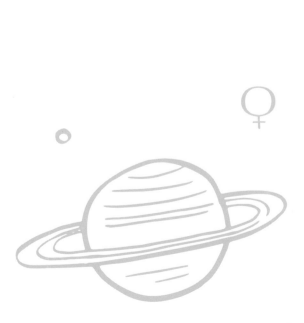

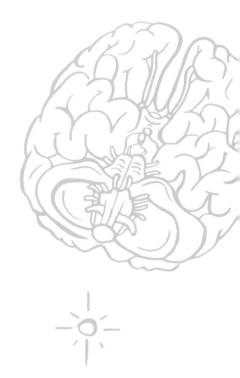

EVERY SIGN IS YOUR SIGN

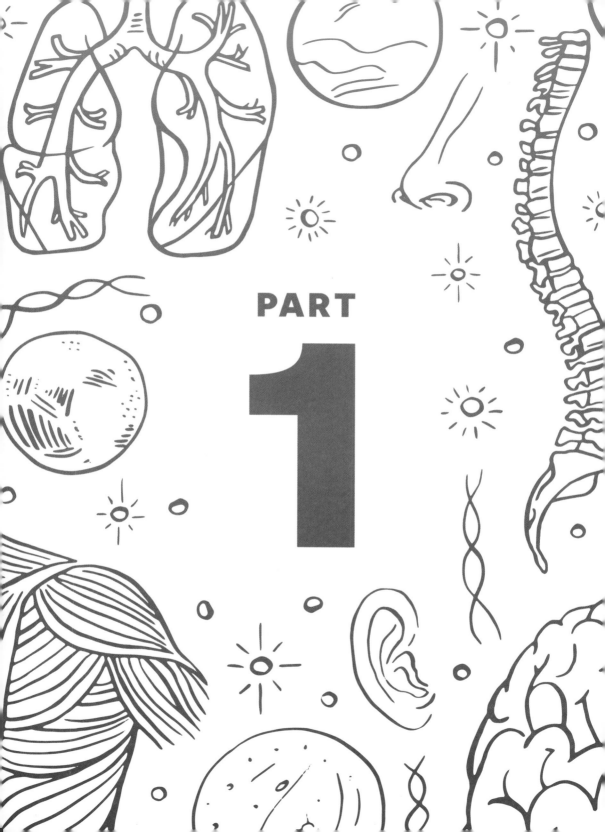

PART

1

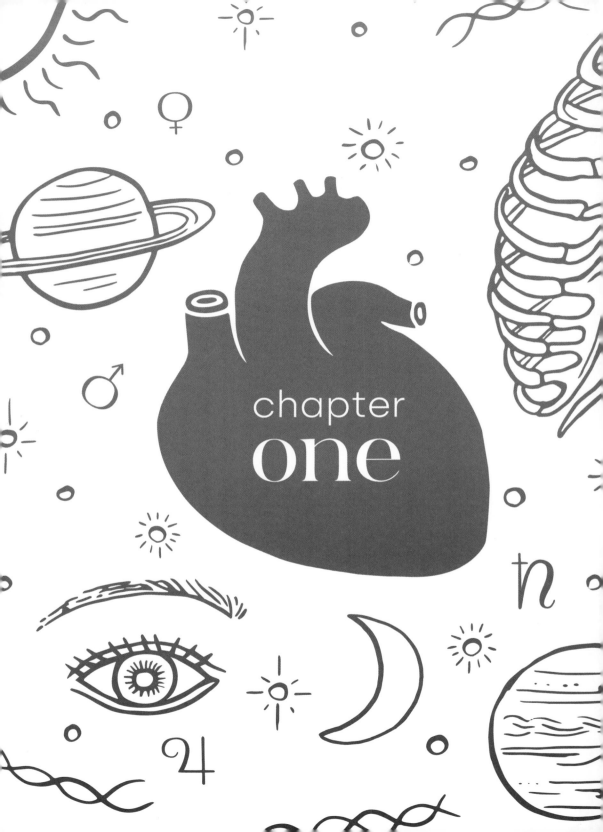

chapter
one

BODY ASTROLOGY BASICS

What do you know about astrology? At the bare minimum, I bet you can tell me what your Sun sign is. And I can feel your fingers itching to flip to the section on your Sun sign. But stop right there! I want this book to be your favorite dog-eared, coffee-stained, cover-ripped resource, and that's simply not going to happen if you flip to one sign and then forget about it. For astrology to work its magic in your life (and for my Virgo dreams to come true), we have some work ahead of us. Make yourself a cup of something and get cozy because I'm about to break a sweat arming you with some real astrological knowledge. My advice is to give this chapter a read first so that then you can knowledgeably flip to your heart's content.

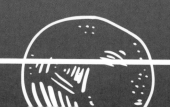

So, what is astrology? I think of it as the observation of planetary patterns and how they correlate with personal patterns. I don't believe planets cause things to happen. Rather, I see astrology as a heavenly mirror for what's already happening. When we know how to read this heavenly mirror, we can each glean more information about our life and how to navigate it. What keeps my trust in astrology, and why I think it continues to resonate with so many others, is its antiquity. Humans have always looked to the sky for some type of information or direction. Some form of astrological practice is found in almost every traditional culture, which is why so many different systems have arisen over time.

Some of the most practiced systems are Western astrology (with roots in ancient Greece, Egypt, Mesopotamia, Arabia, and Europe), Vedic astrology from India, and Chinese astrology or Bazi Suanming. In this book, we're working with Western astrology. There are many differences in these systems (even different zodiacs!), but what they mostly have in common are the planets and interpreting their positions at the time of birth.

Your Sun sign is important, but it's just one part of your astrological genetics. When you were born, all the planets were busy in their travels, moving through various zodiac signs at different speeds. When you took your first breath, it's as though you froze them in time and position, bringing the characteristics, qualities, and energy of their many and unique cosmic locations into your body. This beautiful and complicated snapshot of sky is your astrological anatomy—your birth chart. The Sun is just one dot on the map.

Astrology is complicated (understatement), and it's only natural to chop it up into more palatable pieces. But I need you to know before we move on that most of what we've come to know as astrology is a watered-down quasi-system. I'll do my best to honor the complexity of real astrology while making it easy to understand. This book is even divided into a few boxy pieces for practicality and digestibility. But I'm not going to contribute to the fallacy of Sun sign astrology and let you flounder about, wondering why in the world you don't feel like a Sagittarius. When astrology is chronically taken out of context and reduced to a collection of stereotypes, it loses its usefulness— especially when we apply it to the body. Flipping to your Sun sign's section is taking astrology out of context. Seriously, don't do it yet.

My hope is that after some self-study, you begin to think of every sign as your sign. Sure, the sections on your Sun, Moon, or rising sign may feel more natural to you, but I encourage you to get to know all twelve. If you recognize yourself in an unexpected sign, trust that. I guarantee there's a deeper astrological reason for it. Although they may vary in importance, every single sign is and will always be in your birth chart. So, a sign you've never considered may become, or may already be, a primary player in your health.

Astrology is dynamic. No, you can't change your birth chart, but the planets kept moving after you arrived. As they move, they enliven and activate your chart in new ways. Today's planetary cycles are interacting with your astrological genetics right now, correlating with times of peace, challenge, wellness, and illness. You were born with a unique elemental mixture, or body climate. Today's planetary cycles are like weather patterns, passing over your elemental body, creating new and temporary climates. Mars may parch it. Venus may drench it. So, yes, you may always be a Libra, but depending on what's going on in the sky, your body's needs may be vastly different from what they were years, months, or even days ago.

The Medical Astrology Lens

Medical astrology turns the birth chart into a physical map and tells you about your body's nature. You'll soon learn that each zodiac sign is associated with specific body areas. At the most basic level, the sign positions of the planets at birth tell us about the health of these parts and systems. But the eye trained in medical astrology offers powerful preventative medicine, guiding you on how to keep your unique nature balanced with food, movement, and lifestyle. When illness pops up, the chart can offer information on root cause, proper treatment, and optimal treatment timing. In this book, I use the terms *physical astrology*, *body astrology*, *astro-fitness*, and *astro-nutrition* to describe my food and fitness subspecialty of the craft. Just know that all these variations arise from Western medical astrology.

As a branch of Western astrology, medical astrology has roots in Egypt, Mesopotamia, Arabia, and elsewhere. But its clearest connections may lie in ancient Greece during the Hellenistic period. Humoral theory reigned with physicians believing disease was an imbalance of the four humors of the body (yellow bile, blood, black bile, and phlegm). These four humors were eventually associated with seasons, elements, planets, and zodiac signs, introducing the idea that the time of birth influenced the elemental makeup of the body. At this time, chances were if you were a physician, you were also an astrologer.

So how does astrology tie into your health? It begins with heaven and earth sharing a vocabulary. We're about to describe astrology with terms of the natural world—*temperature, moisture, elements,* and *modes of being.* Everything else in the world can be described in the same way. When we match up these qualities, we discover that every food, movement, medical intervention, herb, supplement, and even flash-in-the-pan wellness trend share an imprint with similar planets or signs. Medical astrology isn't a miracle cure, it's a lens. Once you grasp the foundations, you can apply them to any modern, traditional, or not-yet-created healing modality you wish. If you're interested in the history of medical astrology, a good book to check out would be *Traditional Medical Astrology* by J. Lee Lehman.

The wellness world is a confusing space, and this book isn't meant to be another voice in an already saturated industry. Instead, think of it as a clarifying guide. There's truly no one-size-fits-all approach to health, and astrology only confirms this. My passion, and the purpose of this book, is to teach you how to use astrology to maintain and enhance health and what that means for each of us (because it's certainly not the same). Knowing your personal astrology will help you sift through the voices, making obvious what's for you and what's not. As you get to know your personal astrology, you'll begin to understand what your body truly needs and, more powerfully, you'll receive the confirmation that you knew all along. Here's a crash course in the essentials.

The Qualities

The four qualities—hot, cold, wet, and dry—are universal concepts, but the way we're looking at them here flowers out of Hellenistic thought. To make sense of the celestial, we can use the terrestrial—and vice versa. Earth and sky imitate each other and share a natural vocabulary. Every planet and sign can be broken down into simple qualities such as hot or cold. Every action and experience of the body can be expressed in similar language.

Understanding the qualities can help you sort through what may or may not be medicinal for you. As you choose food, movement, and treatment options for yourself, think about what qualities they will bring into your body and how they may mix with your personal qualities. For example, a "hot" form of exercise may warm a cold body but aggravate a hot body when done too frequently.

Hot: Heat speeds things up. Heat energizes, but too much heat is agitating, inflammatory, and damaging. Excess heat creates dryness.

Cold: Cold slows things down. Too much cold can depress and fatigue the body. Excess cold creates moisture.

Dry: Dryness separates things and brings definition, clarity, and solidity to the body. Too much dryness can stiffen the body and rob it of nutrients, making it withered and deficient.

Moist/Wet/Damp: I use these words interchangeably. Moisture mixes things together and makes the body pliable, soft, and relaxed. Too much moisture burdens the body and erodes its boundaries, making it vulnerable.

The Elements

What qualities are you dominant in? Well, that's going to depend on your unique elemental mix. In astrology, the elements are the physical and non-physical building blocks of the body and psyche. They correlate with the seasons of the year, the seasons of life, the four humors, the lunar phases, the menstrual cycle—the list goes on and on. Although some medical astrologers may use the elemental systems of Ayurveda or Chinese Medicine, in this book I'm using the Hellenistic lens (with a bit of Chinese Medicine thrown in, because I can't help it). It's important to understand that elements from different traditions aren't always one-to-one correlations. Air in Western medical astrology and Air in Ayurveda don't necessarily behave the same.

In Western medical astrology, there are four elements: Fire, Air, Earth, and Water. Each of us has all four in our body, but we are typically dominant in one or two. Which one are you dominant in? You might be surprised to hear that it has almost nothing to do with your Sun sign and more to do with your Moon and rising signs.

Elements are not static but instead transform into one another, just as the seasonal year turns. Their levels in the body naturally rise and fall, but illness occurs when one or more become excessive or deficient. When this happens, opposing and complementary elements can be used to restore balance. Note that the four qualities combine to form the four elements.

Hot + Wet = Air (The Air signs are Gemini, Libra, and Aquarius.)

Hot + Dry = Fire (The Fire signs are Aries, Leo, and Sagittarius.)

Cold + Dry = Earth (The Earth signs are Taurus, Virgo, and Capricorn.)

Cold + Wet = Water (The Water signs are Cancer, Scorpio, and Pisces.)

The Modes

Each element has multiple modes, or ways it can express and move through the world. The three modes are cardinal, fixed, and mutable. For example, there are many modes of Earth—stone, sand, soil, flower, tree, metal, and so on. They're all Earth, but they don't act the same.

Cardinal energy moves directly or forcefully. The cardinal signs are Aries, Cancer, Libra, and Capricorn.

Fixed energy moves consistently. The fixed signs are Taurus, Leo, Scorpio, and Aquarius.

Mutable energy moves flexibly or adaptably. The mutable signs are Gemini, Virgo, Sagittarius, and Pisces.

Taurus, Virgo, and Capricorn may all be Earth signs, but their Earth behaves differently because they have different modes. On the other hand, Gemini, Virgo, Sagittarius, and Pisces may be of different elements, but they have a lot in common because they're all mutable in mode. A sign's mode, or how it moves, becomes particularly important in astrological fitness. Each type of movement is an entire universe, and mode helps us articulate its diversity. The yoga world, for example, is massive; there are so many ways to practice, from relaxed yin yoga to intense ashtanga. Beyond the elements, mode gives us another way to astrologically categorize movement, whether it's various yogic traditions, martial arts lineages, or different types of skiing.

Although I may not mention mode explicitly throughout the book, it's foundational to most of my astro-fitness work. When I'm writing routines, I take a lot of creative cues from a sign's mode. It helps me discern how signs of the same element may move differently or how signs of different elements may move the same. For example, Fire exercise generally has a cardiovascular component, but there are a million ways to do this, and each mode takes a unique approach. Let's use running as an example. Cardinal running might look like a short and gnarly sprint session. Fixed running might look like long, slow distance or working on consistent pacing. And mutable running might take the form of an intuitive interval session or running on variable terrain. Although you may prefer one of these training styles over another, if you want to be a well-rounded runner, chances are you need to work within all three modes.

Astrology Is Not a Diet

As a medical astrologer, the most common question I get is, what type of diet and exercise is best for my zodiac sign? Surprise—I'm not going to teach you how to eat and exercise for your Sun sign in this book. There are many reasons for this, but let's start with the astrological ones. Each zodiac sign is a massive spectrum of possibility. To assume that every Aries across the globe will benefit from the same food and movement is scientifically, energetically, culturally, and astrologically unreasonable. It's not useful to make statements such as all Air signs should be runners or all Water signs should be swimmers. Just like any sign can be a vegetarian, any sign can really dig yoga, weightlifting, or tennis. Perhaps more importantly, each of these activities can be performed in an Aries way, a Taurus way, a Gemini way—you get the picture.

Remember that heaven and earth share a vocabulary. We've described astrology with terms of the natural world—*temperature, moisture, elements,* and *modes of being.* Everything else in the world can be described in the same way. When we match up these qualities, we discover that every type of food and movement shares imprints with signs and planets. So, sure, your chart *might* tell us what types of exercise you're more attracted to or what foods you prefer. But more importantly, your chart tells us how your body assimilates food and movement and may reveal any functional or structural issues that could come up along the way. The birth chart is a little bit like a lab test. It gives us a snapshot of how your body is different from another body. For example, all twelve signs can suffer from digestive issues, but the underlying cause, symptom presentation, other organ systems involved, and healing journey will differ.

Astrology also tells us about your mental-emotional relationship with food and movement—how you think, feel, and talk to yourself and others about food and movement. The birth chart has a unique way of compassionately uncovering any harmful belief systems or societal judgments about eating you've possibly internalized as well as how they may be disrupting your sense of well-being. Throughout the book, I refer to these belief systems as *food talk, food thoughts, food stories, food narratives,* and so on. In my experience, kindly deconstructing these thoughts and healing the food and movement relationship are much more crucial than what you eat or how you move. And it's where my true passion in medical astrology lies.

Within food talk, astrology teaches us to leave room for individuation and refrain from labeling food and movement practices as good, bad, better than, or less than. These terms are not only harmful products of diet and "wellness" culture, but they're irrelevant in body astrology. Because your birth chart is a unique mixture of qualities, your version of "healthy" food and movement will probably look very different from someone dominant in opposing qualities. When we consider how many planetary and elemental combinations are possible at birth, it's clear that a one-size-fits-all approach has no place in body astrology.

Real astrology challenges us to hold polarities maturely. Let me give you a challenging polarity right now: veganism and eating animal protein. Will some signs be attracted to one over the other? Perhaps. But the truth is, every single sign can be a vegan or a meat-eater. In astro-nutrition, foods are energetic tools. For example, both plant and animal foods can be therapeutic for Aries, but for different reasons. One can cool down excess Aries Fire, and one can build up deficient Aries Fire. There's always a greater astrological and physical context. In medical astrology, everything carries an imprint that may be therapeutically necessary depending on the situation.

Therapeutic Gestures

Rather than typecasting a sign into one way of eating or moving, it's more helpful to understand each sign's underlying therapeutic gesture so that we can apply the wisdom of astrology to any health context. By gesture, I mean a sign's essence or energetic signature and how that translates into needs and behavior. Signs are vast bodies of energy that can manifest in a multitude of ways, but these ways share a common gesture. To grasp gesture, we tend to boil it down into keywords. For example, a keyword frequently associated with Libra is *balance*. Balance is a vast concept, a gesture, that can be applied to any type of movement or way of eating. Gestures allow us to be as general or as specific as we like. For example, we can focus on balancing yoga postures or get detailed and work on a specific muscular imbalance. Likewise, we can create a generally balanced meal or address specific mineral imbalances in the body. But where does gesture come from and why is Libra associated with balance? It's a combination of Libra's qualities, element, mode, planetary ruler, and seasonal time of year. It's a lot easier to just say "balance." But knowing where a gesture comes from is important, because it keeps us from blindly regurgitating sign stereotypes and also allows us to apply astrological concepts to very specific, therapeutic contexts.

Astro Vocab: Planetary Ruler

From now on, you're going to see *planetary ruler, ruling planet*, or some variation of the two a lot. Each zodiac sign is ruled by a planet. This planet gives the zodiac sign its characteristics. For example, Sagittarius is ruled by the planet Jupiter. Sagittarius's traits didn't come out of thin air—most of them come from Jupiter. We can learn more about a sign by understanding its planetary ruler. For a list of signs and their ruling planets, see the glossary on page 295.

We'll explore each zodiac sign's therapeutic gestures in detail in their respective sections. You can also find them summarized in the nourishment and movement checklists throughout the book. As you read, it may sound as if I'm saying "Aquarius should do this" and "Scorpio should do that," but what I'm talking about is the gesture, or pure essence of a zodiac sign, not a person. Again, you're a person, not a zodiac sign. You have a complex chart where every sign makes an appearance. Think of your chart like a house or book. Moving and eating for your Sun sign alone is like only living in the bathroom or skipping to the last chapter and missing the good stuff. Plus, your Sun sign doesn't account for how the sky and your body change over time. I believe that to be well-rounded bodies, we need to inhabit each gesture of the zodiacal wheel at the appropriate time (we'll talk about this in chapter 2). Can a sign have more than one gesture? Absolutely. But in my experience, the gestures I've given the signs in this book apply to the majority of people.

The astro-fitness concepts in this book are energetic symbols that can be applied to any movement you enjoy, but as a strength and conditioning coach, I emphasize weight training. I've seen strength training play a pivotal role in many people's healing stories, and it's where I've done my deepest astro-fitness research. You can also think of it this way: Every athlete has a strength coach. Elite figure skaters, boxers, snowboarders, dancers, pitchers, and sprinters all supplement their crafts with strength work. You may not be an elite athlete, but when strength talk comes up, ask yourself how it can support your yoga practice, race time, or whatever movement you love. Don't worry—I've applied astrology to as much movement as I could, including yoga and running. You can also find fitness terms in the glossary and online demos of movements from the book at clairegallagher.co/bodyastro.

Where to Start

The most basic pieces of your birth chart are signs, planets, and houses. Once you get those down, you can play with aspects and transits. Though you may be familiar with these pieces, when thinking about body astrology, they each take on different and specific meanings. You know by now that I'm a fan of all twelve signs, and hopefully you are too! But it's also true that some signs, planets, and parts of your chart will play bigger roles in your health than others. Here, we'll break down the basic parts of the chart and how they work in health. Then we'll look at the areas of your chart that are more likely to manifest physically. These are the sections in part two that you will want to explore first. Keep in mind, the guidance in the sign sections is not exhaustive—there's always more astrology where this came from—but it's a solid starting point. For more guidance on exactly where to start, use the flowchart below. Also consult the flowchart for direction when something new arises in your physical experience. It'll help you narrow down which signs, planets, or parts of your chart are most likely involved.

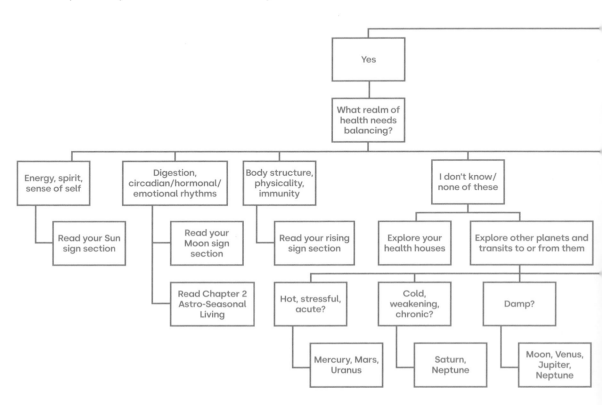

To get the most out of this book, you will need a copy of your birth chart close by. You can get this for free on many websites and apps (see the resources section on page 292 for some of my favorites). To get an accurate chart, you'll not only need your date of birth but also your birthplace and time of birth (as exact as possible!). If you don't know your exact birth time, check your birth certificate or ask a relative. My birth certificate didn't have a time listed and I had to request a long-form certificate from the state. Even if it's an approximation, an educated guess could be the difference between a correct or incorrect Moon and rising sign. I also suggest adjusting the settings of whatever program you're using to display whole sign houses. This is the house system many medical astrologers use and—beginner bonus—it's much easier on the eyes.

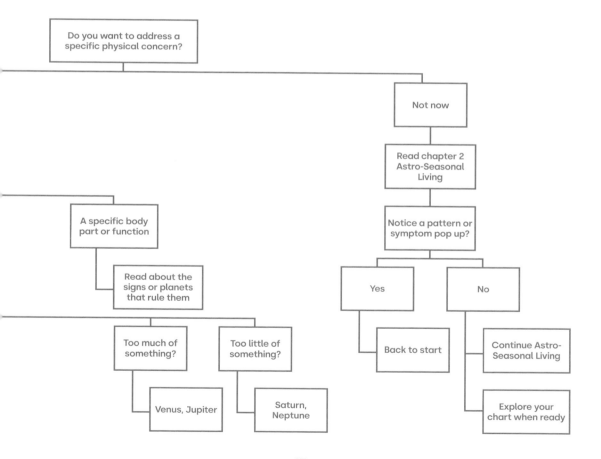

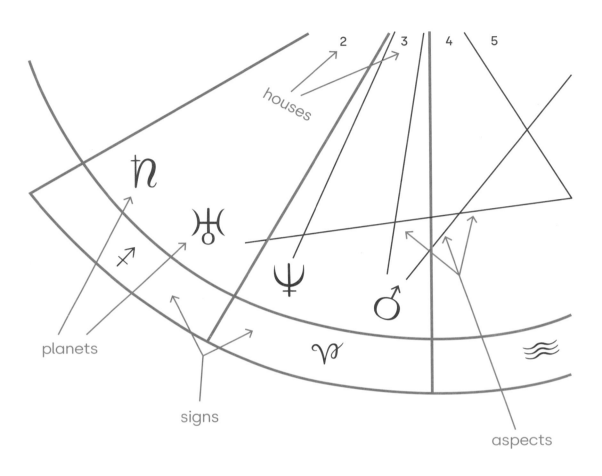

The twelve zodiac signs represent body parts, organs, and systems such as the arms, liver, circulatory system, and so on. The signs receive planetary energy and direct it to a part of the body.

The planets do stuff. They move through the zodiac signs (a.k.a. the body) and create change. In astrology, there are ten planets, including the Sun, Moon, and Pluto. Think of the planets as physiological functions or forces, such as digesting, inflaming, protecting, or connecting—anything with an -ing. Typically, planets are not body parts. They direct or act upon body parts. Pro tip: There are some exceptions to this rule. For example, planets often rule glands because glands initiate function and tell the body what to do.

Astro Vocab: Natal Planet

The birth chart is also known as the natal chart. The planets in your birth chart and their unique locations are your natal planets. For example, we all have Mercury somewhere in our chart, but maybe your Mercury is found in Taurus. That's your natal Mercury. When I put *natal* in front of *any* planet, whether it's Mercury, Saturn, or the Sun, I'm referencing that planet in *your* birth chart. This is an important label as you deepen your astrology practice, because it distinguishes natal planets (planets in your birth chart) from transiting planets, or planets in the sky today.

The twelve houses give us the context of a condition. This is the life area that an imbalance arises from, affects, or is affected by—for example, school, travel, work, or relationships. You can read more about the houses on page 20.

Aspects are the relationships between planets, noted by all the lines in the center of your birth chart. Some common aspects are the conjunction, opposition, square, trine, and sextile, but there are many more. Aspects tell us how planets (a.k.a. body functions) interact with each other. For example, if one of Mars's functions is speeding up and one of Mercury's functions is thinking, we might see some quick wit or even anxiety when they're in relationship with each other. Aspects deserve a book of their own, and we won't spend much time on them here. You can find more information on aspect self-study in the resources section on page 292.

Transits refer to current planetary motion. A transit may tell us about the timing and life cycle of a condition or experience. In my opinion, not everything in your birth chart is active all the time. Different parts of your astrological anatomy become activated and may temporarily alter when planets in the real-time sky pass by (a.k.a. transit) the planets in your chart. Transits are a pivotal part of body astrology because they often change our physical needs. We'll discuss transits in more detail in chapters 2 and 7.

Your Body Astrology Triad

The most basic layer of your personal body astrology is your Sun, Moon, and rising signs. As you read these sections, keep in mind that although you are a mix of all three, they govern different facets of your health. As summarized in the image on page 16, the Sun is more spiritual (as in the life-giving spirit),

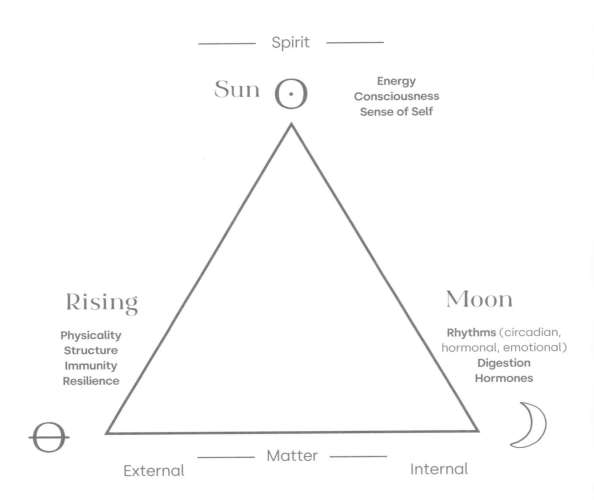

Spirit

Sun ☉

Energy
Consciousness
Sense of Self

Rising

Physicality
Structure
Immunity
Resilience

Moon

Rhythms (circadian,
hormonal, emotional)
Digestion
Hormones

Matter

External   Internal

whereas the Moon and rising signs are more material. You don't need to apply all the information from these sections all at once. Depending on what you desire to heal or improve, you may want to pay closer attention to one over the others for a season. Focus on the one that feels most important right now, and as you get the hang of things, I encourage you to customize your approach. Pick and choose single tips from each section that feel resonant and leave the rest.

If the information in your Sun, Moon, and rising sign sections feels contradictory, remember that they govern different facets of health. It's rarely this black-and-white in practice, but I encourage you to fall back on this lens if you're feeling confused:

Your Sun sign's section may speak more to your psychological and spiritual journey with food and movement instead of the daily nuts and bolts.

Your Moon sign's section may speak more directly to your daily nourishment needs and your unique energy flow.

Your rising sign describes your physicality, and its section may offer insight on keeping your body's structure healthy with movement.

The house locations of your Sun and Moon can also help you discern if one is more of a health priority. Both your Sun and Moon are important physical markers no matter where they are placed in the chart. But if one happens to be in a health house (more on those on page 20), it's probably more important in your personal body astrology than the other.

Also, check your chart for a planet pileup, often called a stellium. These celestial traffic jams are pretty easy to spot and look like a bunch of planets stuck together in one part of the chart. The zodiac sign of this pileup is very important in your physical experience, even if it doesn't include your Sun or Moon. Stelliums are very concentrated areas of planetary energy or life focus, and it's common to feel more like this sign than your Sun sign. If you have a stellium, prioritize that section.

After getting to know your body astrology triad, I suggest learning how the cycles of the Sun and Moon change your movement and nutritional needs throughout the month and year; see chapter 2.

SUN SIGN

I know I stomped all over Sun signs to make a point, but I'm not too proud to backpedal just a smidge. No, your Sun sign isn't everything, but it is that oomph and magic spark that keep you alive. The Sun is your generator, or vital force. We must keep the Sun healthy because if that light goes out—game over.

Beyond being your energy generator, the Sun represents your consciousness, sense of self, and spiritual health. When you're disconnected from yourself, the Sun and its zodiac sign may begin to show physical symptoms. It's just like in real life when clouds block the Sun or when the low light of winter leads to a dip in mood. Deep fatigue, depression, and disinterest in life are clues that the astrological Sun needs some attention.

MOON SIGN	Your Sun and Moon signs work together. The Moon is a receptor and reflector. Its job is to receive and then deliver the Sun's energy to all the bits that need it. The Moon gets energy to where it needs to go. This isn't meant to be esoteric. I'm talking about actual caloric energy. Your Moon sign describes your unique way of using energy. For example, some people operate in spurts, while others have a slow, steady flow. One is not better than the other. Clearly the main way we receive energy is through food, making the Moon a huge player in digestive health. The Moon changes daily and reflects daily rhythms including mood, appetite, fluid levels, workout performance, and hormonal shifts.
RISING SIGN	Your rising sign is the zodiac sign that was coming up over the horizon when you took your first breath. Because the Earth rotates on its axis, the rising sign changes very frequently, approximately every two to three hours depending on the time of year. This is why having an accurate birth time is important. The rising sign is also called the Ascendant sign, or simply the Ascendant.
	Your rising sign describes your body's interface—how it looks, walks, and talks. It's very physical. In psychological astrology, this sign often describes how you present yourself to the world, at work, to acquaintances, or on social media. The rising sign is like a front door, a bouncer, a filter, or packaging. Everything that enters or is applied to the body—light, sound, food, exercise, or pathogen—is met by this sign and its body areas. If we run with this idea, it's easy to see how the rising sign could play a role in immunity and nourishing it may keep the good things in and the bad things out.

Going Deeper

Although essential, your Sun, Moon, and rising signs are just the basic framework of your astrological body. Here, we'll go over some more complex layers of body astrology for you to explore when you're ready. Again, don't try to combine and apply all this information at once. Astrology is as much about timing as anything else, and not everything in your chart is active all the time. You don't experience childhood bumps and bruises at the same time as midlife aches and pains. The chart, just like the body and health experience, unfolds over your lifetime. As you read through the following material, ask yourself if it's a relevant piece or theme for you right now. If it is, flip to that section. If not, come back when and if it becomes relevant later.

MARS AND SATURN

All planets are important health indicators, but for the sake of simplicity, there are some that you really need to pay attention to beyond your Sun and Moon. Mars and Saturn are the most likely to create roadblocks to health. I don't like to think of them as bad planets, but the body has a narrow homeostatic window, and the extreme forces these planets apply can easily push it into imbalance. Mars beams heat. Its conditions are inflammatory, aggravating, agitating, and acute. Saturn beams cold. Its conditions are restricting, concretizing, weakening, and chronic. Know the sign and house location of these planets in your birth chart. Know where they are in the real-time sky and read up on their body associations. Keep an eye on them and use their section's information as a resource for healing and prevention.

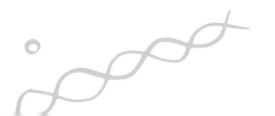

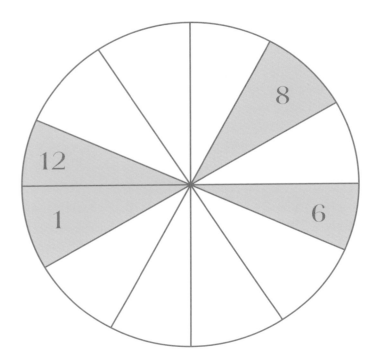

The Health Houses

The houses represent life areas and give us context. There are only twelve houses, but any life experience you can imagine falls into one. Although any house can interplay with health, the first, sixth, eighth, and twelfth houses highlighted in the image above are directly health related. A house doesn't necessarily tell us where in the body a health issue is (that's a zodiac sign's job) but may reveal its nature and the nature of our experience with it. The zodiac signs on these houses and any planets in these houses are important to pay attention to. They may represent body parts (signs) or functions (planets) that are, or may become, a part of your health story. For example, maybe your Sun, Moon, and rising signs are all Fire and Air, but you learn that you have Venus in Cancer in the sixth house of daily health. The body areas of Cancer should definitely be on your astrology radar. It's likely that the fluidic and hormonal experiences so common for this placement are something you deal with regularly.

Pro tip: You don't have to have a planet in a health house for that house to be important. Even if a house appears "empty," it's still a part of your life. The zodiac sign on that house will give you more information about it. Plus, planets in the current sky will travel through your health houses many times throughout your life.

THE FIRST HOUSE: WHOLE BODY

How the houses are divided is and will always be a hot debate in astrology. But regardless, the first house and the rising sign will coincide. They're both beginnings, and the health attributes we gave to the rising sign are shared by the first house. The sign on and any planets in your first house speak about your visible, tangible body; its resilience and vitality; and how it interfaces with the world. The nutrition and fitness sections in this sign's section may come naturally to you. Or they could be used as tools to boost vitality when you're feeling depleted or to restore your boundaries when you're feeling physically or emotionally invaded.

THE SIXTH HOUSE: DAILY BODY

The sixth house is the house of daily body care and preventative medicine. Although larger accidents and illnesses can be associated with the sixth house, in practice I find it more common for any issues here to be run-of-the-mill daily aggravations. But these can certainly add up and become something more serious over time, which is exactly why we need daily sixth-house care and why the body areas belonging to the corresponding sign need regular attention. The sign on this house and its section may offer you guidance on your daily self-care priorities, habits, and routines.

THE EIGHTH HOUSE: CHRONIC BODY

Eighth house health conditions can be more intense or long-term, possibly requiring treatment or surgery or posing a potential financial or emotional burden. Eighth house conditions are transformative, crucible-like, and often ripe with psychological suffering. Not to scare anyone, but if you've had a near-death experience, that's eighth house stuff. Death, birth, survival, purification, and regeneration are major themes here. Eighth house health stories may act as a transformational doorway. The health crisis that brought me to astrology was a combined eighth and twelfth house experience. I felt stripped to nothing, but the hidden gem was that I was forced (because I was too weak to do otherwise) to submit to the unexpected process and path that was unfolding in front of me. Even if I'm never 100 percent, the lessons I learned and the life choices I made because of my illness truly made me *me*. It gave me the tools, felt experience, and compassion to do what I do now. And this book wouldn't exist without it.

This type of story is not unique to me. If you are dealing with a chronic condition, try to befriend your eighth house. Its sign or resident planets may offer insight about the root cause and other body systems to explore in treatment, as well as any underlying mental-emotional patterns, societal or familial conditioning, or even subconscious themes to explore as part of your healing. Even if you don't have an eighth house condition, use the suggestions in its corresponding sign section as an occasional tune-up, just to make sure this part of your astro-anatomy is happy and functioning.

THE TWELFTH HOUSE: HIDDEN BODY

In traditional astrology, the twelfth house is associated with places and experiences of confinement—whether positive or negative—such as monasteries, ashrams, hospitals, institutions, and prisons. When we apply this broad idea to the body, any health conditions that arise from the twelfth house are often isolating in nature. It could be an experience that separates you from friends, society, and life as usual, or it could be something intimate and close to your heart that you simply don't share. This house doesn't often see the light of day, and it rules the hidden realms of health such as sleep, spirituality, and sometimes sexual and mental health.

Because of its hiddenness, there's also an essence of mystery to these experiences. Conditions rooted here are often hard to understand, changeable, and perhaps even misdiagnosed or mistreated. It's also the house of self-sabotage, getting in your own way and the subconscious reflected in the body. Sometimes we perpetuate these conditions, knowingly or unknowingly, with our thoughts and actions. For maintenance, use the suggestions in your twelfth house's corresponding sign section as an occasional compassionate light that you shine on this realm just to make sure all's well.

Transits

Your chart gets activated in new ways as the current sky changes. These are called transits. The image on page 23 shows how transits are typically displayed on a birth chart. Your natal planets are inside the wheel, while the transiting planets move around them on the outside. I like to think of transits as astrological seasons. We explore the general seasons of the Sun and Moon and how to align with them in chapter 2. But lengthier transits often coincide with significant personal and physical changes and may present new nutritional, movement, or self-care needs. In part three, we identify transits to or from all the planets and the lifestyle tweaks they may require.

If your natal Sun, Moon, or rising sign is currently being transited by a planet (especially a slow one, such as Saturn, Uranus, Neptune, or Pluto), focus on the sections of the signs and planets involved. These parts of your

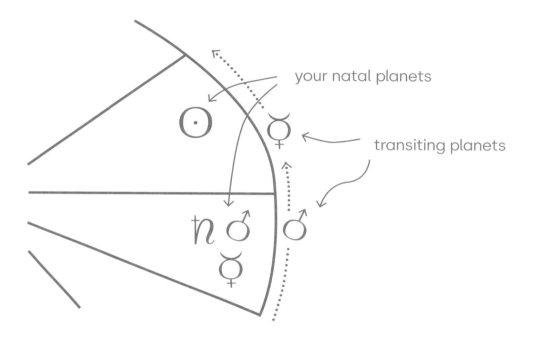

your natal planets

transiting planets

astro-anatomy probably need some love. This goes for other planets in your chart too, beyond the Sun and Moon. For example, maybe you're a Gemini Sun, Sagittarius Moon, and Gemini rising, but Neptune is transiting your natal Venus in Pisces. This will bring Venus, Neptune, and Pisces health themes to the surface for a handful of years. In this case, I suggest either incorporating or fully focusing on the information in the Venus, Neptune, and Pisces sections. To know what transits you're currently experiencing, you'll need an astrology program, app, or personalized almanac. See the resources section for some of my favorites.

Becoming Your Own Body Astrologer

When I say every sign is your sign, what I really mean is every sign is your *tool*. You just need to know when and how to use them. When you know the basic dynamics between the elements, signs, and planets, you can use the food, movement, and other healing tools in their sections to restore balance. You may always be a Taurus Sun or a Sagittarius Moon, but if those parts of your astrological anatomy become imbalanced, it's likely you'll need to call on other parts of the zodiac to help you out. Sometimes a Taurus problem needs Taurus therapeutics, but sometimes it needs Scorpio, Virgo, or Aquarius therapeutics. These therapeutic relationships are the basis of astro-medicine. If your astrology brain isn't too full yet, here's a few basic techniques for using them.

Elemental Balancing

Each sign and planet is associated with an element (see the master list in appendix A). Although your body may be dominant in one or two, it's important to understand how all four elements interrelate. Remember, when there's too much or too little of an element, we can experience symptoms. For example, too much Water might create gut issues and sadness. The Fire tools from the Aries, Leo, or Sagittarius sections could dry things up. Elements generate and control each other. When one increases, another decreases. To restore your body's element balance, you can use opposing or complementary elements. As seen in the chart on page 25, there are many elemental relationships, but the foundation is that Fire and Water balance each other, while Air and Earth balance each other. This is a symbolic way of looking at the body, but its translation is very physical. For example, we might want to anchor Air when it's anemic. We might want to feed Fire when it's depressed. We might want to boil Water when it's infected. You can find a detailed introduction to each element at the beginning of its chapter.

Fire	Air	Earth	Water
Increases Fire	Fans Fire	Feeds Fire	Extinguishes Fire
Brightens Air	Increases Air	Anchors Air	Humidifies Air
Enlivens Earth	Lightens Earth	Increases Earth	Softens Earth
Boils Water	Evaporates Water	Holds Water	Increases Water

Zodiac Balancing

Elemental balancing is a great place to start, but if you want to get more specific, you can take a similar approach with zodiac signs. Just like elements, zodiac signs have relationships too. If you're a visual person, you can learn a lot about sign relationships by looking at your chart and seeing which signs are across from or at angles to each other. Cosmic energy never acts in a vacuum. When something happens on one side of the wheel, it affects the other side, and so on. There are many types of sign relationships, but I find sign pairs to be the most important.

SIGN PAIRS

Sign pairs sit exactly 180 degrees across from each other in the birth chart. These are often referred to as *polarities*, but I prefer *pairs*, because my goal is to get these signs to work as a team instead of acting like a seesaw.

Aries and Libra	Cancer and Capricorn
Taurus and Scorpio	Leo and Aquarius
Gemini and Sagittarius	Virgo and Pisces

Although these signs may be considered opposites in popular astrology, in medical astrology their body systems need to work together. When they aren't working together, we see conditions of excess (too much) or deficiency (too little). For example, too much Taurus energy might express as constipation. We could try bringing in the tools of its sign pair, Scorpio, to relieve it. Or suppose you're a Libra Sun who struggles with unstable blood sugar (a pretty common Libra complaint). The nutrition suggestions in the Libra section could certainly help you out, but so could the high protein consumption referenced in the Aries section.

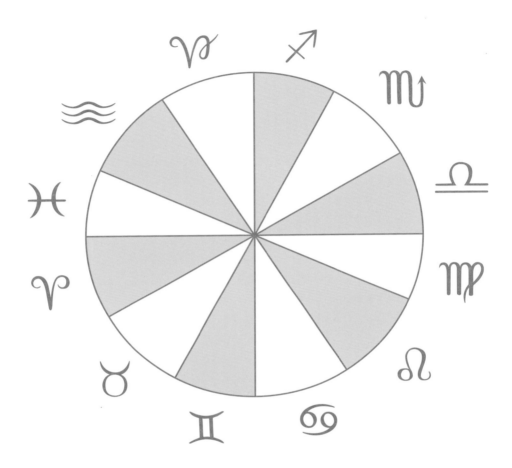

Here's a more complicated example using transits: Let's pretend a lot of planets are currently moving through Capricorn. Your chart doesn't have any planets in Capricorn, but you're a Cancer Moon. Because these signs are paired, the planets traveling through Capricorn can beam their energy across the cosmic street and affect your Cancer Moon. In this case, you might want to give the Capricorn section a look for any applicable tweaks to your self-care approach.

Creating Your Own Cosmic Cures

As you go forward in your body astrology journey, my hope is that you become your own astrological authority. Ancient texts and books are great, and teachers are fabulous, but with this book you have everything you need to make your own astrologically informed self-care decisions. You don't need some-one to tell you stinging nettle, chili powder, and that sprint workout are all ruled by Mars. Because you know Mars, you can make your own assessment.

No matter how cutting-edge or ancient, all food, movement, and healing practices can be evaluated through an astrological lens. Remember, heaven, earth, and the body all share a vocabulary. When we know the essence of a planet, sign, and therapeutic, we can match them up with confidence and use the basic principles of astrological healing to apply them.

Here are a few guiding questions to get you started. In the list below, the word *therapeutic* is meant to encompass anything remotely related to healing—food, supplement, herb, homeopathic remedy, movement, medical intervention, appointment, and more.

✦ Is this therapeutic hot, cold, wet, or dry? Which signs or planets share these qualities?

✦ Does this therapeutic use Fire, Air, Earth, or Water, or remind me of an element in some way? Which signs and planets share this element?

✦ Which parts or functions of the body is this therapeutic targeting? Which signs or planets rule them?

✦ What type of symptoms does this therapeutic address? Which signs or planets tend to experience them?

✦ How does this therapeutic make me feel? Which signs or planets does this remind me of?

✦ What macro- or micronutrient makes up the bulk of this food? Which planet or sign rules it?

✦ Are the timing and application of this therapeutic slow, fast, intermittent, cyclical, intuitive, or tightly regulated? Which signs or planets does this remind me of?

✦ Does this therapeutic act in a cardinal, fixed, or mutable way? Does this therapeutic address a condition that's more cardinal, fixed, or mutable? Which signs also operate this way?

✦ Is this therapeutic more physical, emotional, mental, or spiritual? Which signs or planets also work on these planes?

✦ What is the desired outcome of this therapeutic? (Example: to soothe, build, connect, soften, protect, strengthen, energize.) Which planet also desires to do this?

✦ What does this therapeutic look like, taste like, smell like, feel like? How and where does this therapeutic grow? What signs or planets does this remind me of?

✦ What types of people are typically attracted to this therapeutic? Which cosmic players do they remind me of?

Before You Flip!

Take a breath and come on back to planet Earth. That was a lot of information! One of the biggest lessons I've learned while being a consulting astrologer is that the most complex information is not always the most healing information. Usually—and especially when it comes to the body—starting small and doing one thing at a time is the most profound. Begin with your body astrology triad or the seasonal recommendations in chapter 2 and gradually work your way deeper. Again, there's no wrong way to do this, and you have plenty of time. A few words of wisdom before you go:

✦ Just because a condition is on a list does *not* mean you've had, have, or will have it. And likewise, just because a food or movement modality is on a list does *not* mean you should or shouldn't eat it or do it. There are no rules in this book. Use your common sense and internal wisdom, and remember that real astrology is vast. When in doubt, always ask a professional.

✦ As you've already read, I use the words *imbalance*, *excess*, and *deficiency* frequently. This comes directly from my experience and education in Chinese Medicine, where this terminology is commonplace. These words are not meant to imply that something is wrong with you or that you are lacking in any way. They're simply the most straightforward way to categorize this rather complex information.

✦ The main material in each zodiac sign section applies to that sign in any context, whether it's your Sun, Moon, or rising sign, or if it's identified as a significant player in your health for another reason. Other planets in that sign are briefly mentioned at the end of each section.

✦ You'll notice that Pluto is missing. I left out Pluto because it should be handled with professional care. It takes a little over twenty years for Pluto to move through one zodiac sign, which means everybody born within a few years of you probably has Pluto in the same place. This means it's probably not very personal to you unless it meets very specific criteria. Pluto can be a massive health player, but this is usually only the case when it's in a very tight and uncomfortable relationship (aspect) with one of your vital health planets by birth or transit. And even then, it's not guaranteed to express at all.

Pluto may or may not correlate with life-altering illnesses and events—births, deaths, surgeries, healings, or other significant experiences. Pluto seems to do its work by deconstructing something and then reconstructing it, whether it's a body part or a career. But having everybody read about Pluto in Libra, Scorpio, Sagittarius, or Capricorn would probably cause more unwarranted astrological harm than good.

Even though I included them, keep this same wisdom at your fingertips when reading about the other outer planets, Uranus and Neptune.

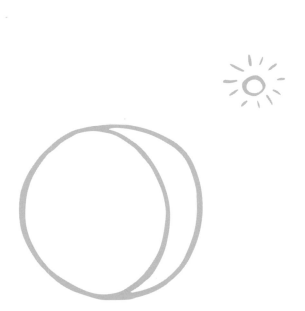

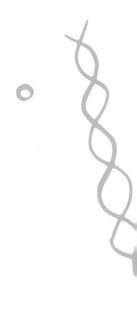

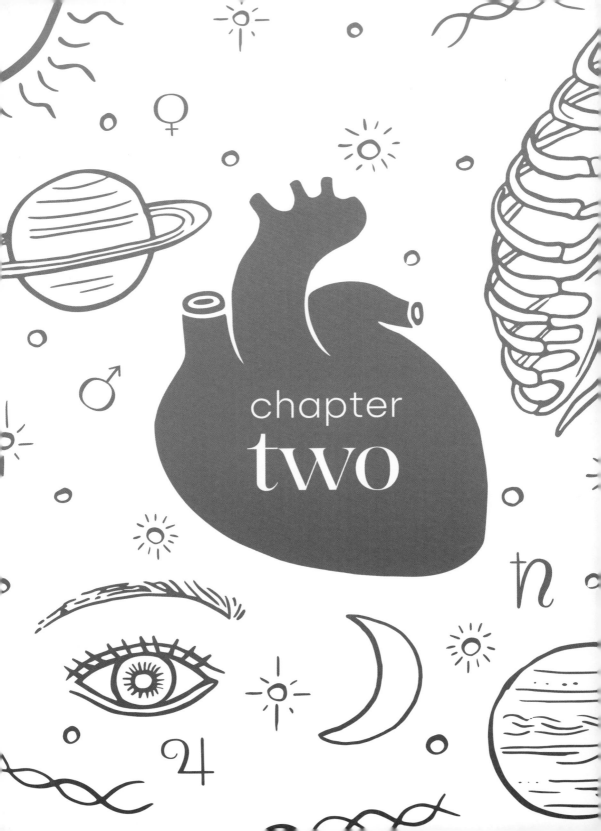

chapter
two

ASTRO-SEASONAL LIVING

In chapter 1, we talked extensively about the pieces of your birth chart. This complex chart is the celestial body programming you were born with. Every experience you have, food you eat, and workout you do gets filtered through this celestial grid. It shows how you receive, process, think, and feel about food and movement. It uncovers strengths and any blocks to nourishment that could come up throughout your journey. And this is just the foundation. Your birth chart may never change, but thanks to the shifting astrological seasons, you certainly do. In astro-nutrition and astro-fitness, your chart and the changing astrology are layered to create a nourishment practice that's physically supportive and cosmically aligned at any stage of life.

Astro-Seasonal Layering

Solar and Other Planetary Cycles

(a.k.a. transits)

How my food and movement needs change throughout the year and beyond.

Lunar Cycle

How my food and movement needs change throughout the month.

Birth Chart

How I think and feel about food and movement.

How my body receives and processes food and movement.

Physical strengths, weaknesses, and blocks to nourishment.

Cosmic alignment isn't a far-out idea. It's an extension of seasonal living. Astrology is just another way of marking time, but instead of four seasons, we have many more—the twelve solar seasons (or signs), the lunar phases, and other planetary cycles—that create seasons lasting from days to decades. As the planets move through their seasons (also called transits), your chart gets activated in new ways, and the elemental profile of your body shifts in response, presenting new physical and emotional needs. This is why you may always be a Gemini but your tastes, desires, and bodily experience change over time.

But how do we layer the astrological seasons on top of the birth chart? When I'm in a deeper time of healing, I may need my nutrition, movement, and self-care to reflect my birth chart more specifically. But most of the time, unless I'm having a long-term transit or feeling unwell, I keep things simple and live in accordance with the real-time Sun and Moon—what I call astro-seasonal living. I find this to be great health maintenance, and I suggest the same approach for most of my clients. Just as eating seasonal produce gives your body the nutrients it needs to stay healthy during that time of year, eating for the astrological season is that much more potent. This applies to fitness as well. Moving in accordance with the astrological season gives your body the exercise stimulus it's ready to use and integrate.

Astro-seasonal living is also a fantastic way to begin to understand your birth chart. This was actually how I did things when I was first getting into astrology. I was overwhelmed by my chart, but the Sun and Moon felt friend- lier and more accessible. Just by observing their cycles and how my body responded, I learned so much about my chart and the rest of the zodiac. Now I know my birth chart like the back of my hand and intuitively adjust my nourishment routine as needed. These seasons aren't haphazard; they repeat systematically. As you observe them month after month, year after year, you'll gather a ton of empirical data about your birth chart—no astrologer required.

Here, we'll go through the cycles of the Sun and Moon and how they change our needs throughout the months. In part three, we explore the seasons of other planets.

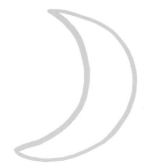

Therapeutic Gesture Wheel*

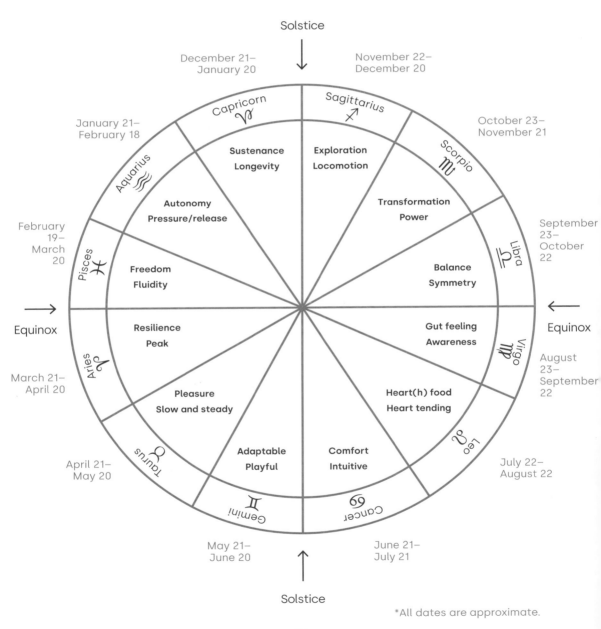

Solstice

December 21–
January 20

November 22–
December 20

January 21–
February 18

October 23–
November 21

Capricorn

Sagittarius

Scorpio

Sustenance
Longevity

Exploration
Locomotion

Aquarius

Transformation
Power

February
19–
March
20

Autonomy
Pressure/release

September
23–
October
22

Pisces

Freedom
Fluidity

Balance
Symmetry

Libra

Equinox

Resilience
Peak

Gut feeling
Awareness

Equinox

Aries

Virgo

March 21–
April 20

August
23–
September
22

Pleasure
Slow and steady

Heart(h) food
Heart tending

Leo

Taurus

Adaptable
Playful

Comfort
Intuitive

April 21–
May 20

July 22–
August 22

Gemini

Cancer

May 21–
June 20

June 21–
July 21

Solstice

*All dates are approximate.

Solar Seasons

We're skipping a ton of astronomy here, but for the purposes of this book, a solar season lasts approximately thirty days. In Western tropical astrology (*tropical* refers to the zodiac we're using), the signs don't correspond with constellations, even though they're named after them. (Sorry, I hope your brain didn't just implode.) Instead, they're based on the positional relationship between the Earth and the Sun. The solstices and equinoxes are the turning points of the astro-seasonal wheel. The sign of Aries begins at the March equinox and extends for thirty days after that point. Then Taurus season begins. When the Sun is in Aries, it's Aries season. When the Sun is in Taurus, it's Taurus season, and so on.

As the Sun moves through each sign during the astrological year, that sign's body areas and health themes are highlighted. Remember the therapeutic gestures from chapter 1? If we superimpose each sign's gestures on an astrology wheel, like the image on page 34, we now have a celestial self-care calendar. For the next month, you have a potent opportunity to use the Sun's light to bring awareness and healing to that area. No matter if you're a Sagittarius or a Cancer, in astro-seasonal living, you're invited to give some attention to Pisces nourishment, movement, and body areas in Pisces season. You can read about each sign's therapeutic gestures in detail in their respective sections.

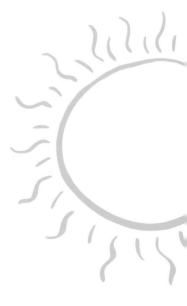

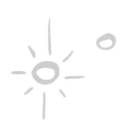

Basic Lunar Phases

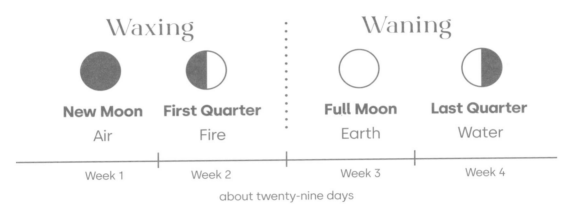

Waxing | Waning

New Moon	First Quarter		Full Moon	Last Quarter
Air	Fire		Earth	Water
Week 1	Week 2		Week 3	Week 4

about twenty-nine days

Lunar Seasons

By lunar seasons I simply mean the phases of the Moon cycle. A few basics: The lunar calendar and our monthly calendar aren't the same. A lunar month is counted from New Moon to New Moon and typically lasts twenty-nine days, although it varies throughout the year. There are many ways to divide the lunar month, but for health, I find it most helpful to divide it into the four major phases illustrated above. This way, each major phase lasts roughly one week, giving every week of the month a theme. We'll unpack these themes later on in the chapter.

I like to think of the Moon phase as a volume knob, reflecting how loud and busy life may be, how much activity we might be able to take on, and our emotional and physical capacity. The Moon phase increases and decreases our energetic capacity. When ignored, we often under- or overexert. Keeping in its rhythm makes us good stewards of our energy. Each lunar phase is also associated with an element. You'll learn more about these elements as you read through part two. As the Moon moves through its phases, the elemental makeup of our body shifts in response. This changes our nourishment needs throughout the month.

But the Moon doesn't just have phases. Like the Sun, it also travels through the twelve signs, although at a much faster pace. The Sun takes one year to travel the wheel, while the Moon only takes one month, staying in each sign for about two and a half days. The sign that the Moon is in gives the day a particular mood or flavor. Staying with our music example, the Moon sign is like a song or music genre, while the Moon phase turns the volume of that song up or down. For example, you can play death metal very softly (perhaps a Scorpio New Moon) or blast your neighbors out with raging classical (perhaps a Libra Full Moon).

Pro tip: You can also use the gesture wheel on page 34 with the Moon instead of the Sun. For example, for the two and a half days the Moon is in Libra each month, focus on the Libra therapeutic gestures. Then when it moves into Scorpio, focus on the Scorpio gestures. But over the years, I've found it more helpful from a health perspective to keep things simple and focus on the solar season and the lunar phase.

Embracing Your Cyclicality

In body astrology, the Moon rules our rhythms. Out of all the planets, its frequent fluctuations most closely mirror our physical ebbs and flows. It's human nature to wax and wane, but somewhere along the way, many of us picked up the idea that fluctuating moods and energy levels aren't normal or healthy. Modern culture disregards our cyclicality and expects us to show up for life statically, as though we're the same day after day. We tend to take this on and expect ourselves to produce and perform constantly. But gradual crescendos and decrescendos are completely normal and even protect our health. It's important to honor our ebbs as much as we honor our flows. The lower points in our energy cycle are what fuel the higher points and vice versa.

The Moon also governs our ability to digest, which goes beyond food and includes anything we ask the body to process, such as emotion, stress, or exercise. The current Moon phase reflects how much stress, whether positive or negative, we're able to process at a given time without moving into discomfort. This is what I mean by energetic capacity. For example, you may feel totally ready for your work presentation under a First Quarter Moon, while that same presentation may feel next to impossible at the end of the lunar cycle.

Movement is another form of stress and is only supportive if our body can "digest" and assimilate it. We don't want to overwhelm the body with too much of anything, even "good" things. Overdoing it creates a traffic jam of hormones and waste products, blocking the body's chance to recover and rebuild. On the other hand, if we don't apply enough stress, we may not experience the positive benefits of exercise. Some days we're primed to receive extreme challenge; other days, a maintenance dose; and others, deep rest. The Moon phase can help us decipher this.

When we reject our cyclical nature, our nourishment routines tend to lack this intelligent cyclicality too. This is when rigid dieting or compulsive exercising may take hold. Chronically rejecting rhythm is where health begins to break down. Paying attention to astrological rhythms can make you more perceptive of and compassionate toward the rhythms within you. This is one of the many reasons why I continuously encourage you to look past "your sign" and understand how the daily astrology impacts your needs.

Side story: Something that used to make my blood boil when I was going through my illness was the phrase "listen to your body." My body felt untrustworthy and uncomfortable to live in. How could it possibly tell me what I needed? Illness or no, most of us are taught to suppress our body's voice from an early age. This is compounded by harmful, biased, and unrealistic media images of the "healthy" ideal. I fell in love with astrology because it helped me rebuild a trust-filled relationship with my body. The Moon's waxing and waning gave me a compassionate framework to follow as I got reacquainted with my body's voice and preferences. This is what I hope for you too. And so, in the following pages, I don't tell you exactly what to eat or how to exercise under each lunar phase. Instead, I've kept things open so that you can invest in your own voice and apply the concepts to whatever food and movement you love.

Myth Buster: Waxing and Waning

Before we explore how your food and movement needs change under each lunar phase, I want you to memorize this: waxing and waning do not equal hard and easy. Instead of being a measure of difficulty, waxing and waning indicate what kind of exercise stimulus your body is ready to receive. By exercise stimulus, I don't mean the type of exercise, such as Pilates versus running, but the *intention* of your session and the outcome it creates. The body under a waxing Moon needs filling up. To meet this need, waxing exercise aims to build up the body. The body under a waning Moon is starting to prepare for the next cycle. To meet this need, waning exercise creates release and makes space. But both can be done in a high- or low-intensity way.

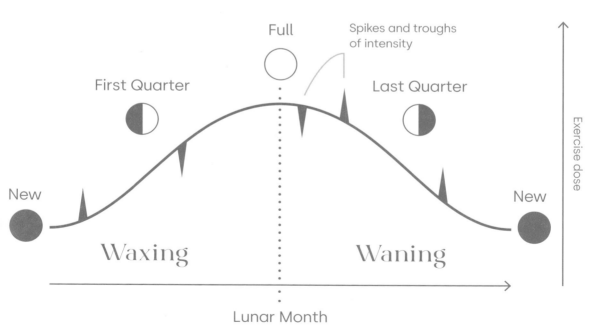

The lunar movement cycle takes on a bell-shaped curve, surging at the waxing gibbous, full, and waning gibbous phases and retreating gradually at either end. So, sure, we may be able to take on an extra session or engage with high intensity more frequently under the Full Moon, but it's not that simple. As shown in the image on page 39, there are several spikes and troughs within each cycle. This is because there's so much more going on in the cosmos, and our bodies, besides the Moon phase. The Moon moves through zodiac signs rapidly, and it's always reflecting the energy of other planets. So, although we're riding this general bell-shaped curve, we're always going to engage with bouts of high or low intensity along the way.

To really understand lunar fitness and nutrition, you have to embody it. Let's go through the four major phases of the lunar cycle and identify their nourishment intentions.

The Lunar Body Cycle

No matter what type of food and movement you prefer, use these guidelines as gentle tweaks or focusing points for each week of the lunar cycle. Remember that lunar weeks and calendar weeks don't sync up perfectly. I use the exact day of the New, First Quarter, Full, or Last Quarter Moon as the beginning of my lunar week. For example, one lunar week begins on the day of the New Moon and spans until the First Quarter Moon, no matter if that "week" lasts five days or nine days.

If you're working with a trainer or other exercise professional and aren't in control of your own exercise programming, not to worry. Simply keep the current phase's intention in mind as you go to your training session or group class. Adjust your mindset and self-talk, and make subtle movement adjustments to honor where you are in the cycle. How you feel immediately, several hours, and twenty-four hours post-workout is vital information about that workout's alignment with your current physical state and the lunar phase. In each section I've listed some keywords to describe how you'd ideally feel after a phase-aligned workout.

New Moon Week

Includes Waxing Crescent

Element: Air (blood; nervous and respiratory systems)

Theme: Set the tone

The New Moon phase is the beginning of the waxing cycle, but it's common to feel not quite ready to begin again at full speed. New cycles are never initiated in a vacuum. They're generated from the resources and experiences left from the cycle before. On the New Moon, the body's energy, fluids, and resources are typically at their lowest because they've been spent waxing, waning, and living during the previous month. Even if you've managed your energy wisely, you may feel as though you have a little less bandwidth. It's important to honor this and to go at your own pace. Keeping in sync with the New Moon phase may be the most important, because it sets the tone for the rest of the month. The most common way we tend to get out of sync with the New Moon is by engaging with movement, dietary, or work extremes. But when we respect this part of the month, we regenerate everything we need to live this new cycle to the fullest.

NEW MOON MOVEMENT

Aim to feel: Revived

During New Moon week, we're laying a supportive foundation for the movement month ahead. New Moon movement is all about pacing. If we do too much too soon, we risk fizzling out at the Full Moon, when we might otherwise feel like doing more frequent or higher-intensity exercise. Complete rest may feel the most appropriate during the hours or days surrounding the exact New Moon. But as the Moon gains size, gradually reintroduce movement that feels reviving and boosts your mood. New Moon movement may create a light sweat and elevate your heart and breath rate, but if someone were to ask you a question while you're moving, you'd ideally be able to respond in a full sentence. With my strength clients, I often describe this as working at a maintenance level—meaning it's worthwhile work but you're not at your threshold. Instead of focusing solely on speed or intensity, explore playful movement, the mind-muscle connection, or developing new skills. But if you feel like hitting a high-intensity session during New Moon week, go for it! You can sprinkle high-intensity peaks and low-intensity ebbs into your routine whenever you want. If it refreshes your body and mind and encourages your spirit, you're right on track.

NEW MOON NUTRITION

Aim to feel: Fortified

Until the Waxing Crescent Moon appears, the New Moon sky is dark and empty, reflecting a need to add back to ourselves. Prepare your body for the cycle ahead with foods and eating patterns that feel stabilizing and substantial. Don't skimp on nourishment. When your body asks for food, give it what it needs without question or guilt. If we don't intentionally fill the New Moon's emptiness with something sustaining, it may be filled by something less supportive later in the cycle—overwork, stress, a pathogen, disordered eating and exercising behaviors, and so on. The New Moon is associated with Air and corresponds with the nervous system. At the start of this week, the body's resources are at their lowest and the nerves need to be "rebuilt." We want our food to act as a soothing anchor for this system as we pick up speed and set the tone for the cycle ahead. Honoring hunger signals is foundational nervous system self-care. Use the New Moon phase as an opportunity to reacquaint yourself with and respect these signals. Keep in mind that New Moon hunger signals may include poor concentration, light-headedness, anxiety, clumsiness, and body weakness.

It's a common misconception that the New Moon is the best time for all things "new," but that's not always the case. Anything involving removal or restriction is inherently out of sync with the New Moon's energetics. Using the New Moon to kick-start dieting or compulsive exercising is misguided. Rather, the New Moon mindset is about what we can *add* to our life to fortify the body and increase our sense of well-being.

First Quarter Moon Week

Includes Waxing Gibbous

Element: Fire (metabolism; muscular and cardiovascular systems)

Theme: Build momentum

The Quarter Moons may be my favorite parts of the lunar cycle. Each Quarter Moon serves as a checkpoint or a crossroads between the New and Full Moons, giving us an opportunity to take personal inventory and adjust course if necessary. The First Quarter Moon is like a crescendo, gradually increasing in size and momentum on its way to fullness. Ideally, the body's resources are refreshed and ready to build on the foundation laid during the New Moon. If you don't feel the slight quickening of this fiery phase, it's a clue that you may not have given yourself enough rest or nourishment during the New Moon phase. On the other hand, look out for taking too much action. During this phase, especially toward the end, it's easy to blur the line between healthy Fire and stress or inflammation.

FIRST QUARTER MOON MOVEMENT

Aim to feel: Strong

During First Quarter Moon week, you may feel ready to add a bit more heat and challenge to the movement patterns established under the New Moon. This phase sends a lot of energy to the muscular and cardiovascular systems, meaning they're often ready and willing to work. At the gym, this might mean lifting heavier, lifting more (a.k.a. increasing your total volume with more sets), or throwing in a conditioning session or two. If you're a runner, upping your mileage or incorporating speed work may feel right. If you're a yogi, consider infusing more heat into your practice with a warm room or a more vigorous flow. Or simply increase your exercise frequency if that feels supportive. As the Moon enlarges, you may desire to flirt with your personal exercise thresh-old more frequently, but be smart about it, because the Full Moon is still on the way. Hard work can feel good, even pleasant, under this phase. But try to treat your movement practice like kindling—something that creates energy and passion for the other parts of your life.

FIRST QUARTER MOON NUTRITION

Aim to feel: Energized

Under the First Quarter Moon, the body's Fire is waking up and needs to be fed and maintained so that it can carry us through the Full Moon and beyond. Life is busier, we may be moving more, and our metabolism is almost at its celestial peak. If we don't give ourselves enough food during this phase, we may feel more stressed, less resilient, and could be heading for a Full Moon crash. Slightly different from the heavy, restorative focus of New Moon food, our focus now is to keep the body and mind quick and agile. Focus on foods and feeding patterns that feel energizing. Classic hunger signals like a gnawing stomach are more common under this phase, but irritability, headache, sweating, muscle twitches, and even heart palpitations are all First Quarter cues to stop and eat. Use the First Quarter phase as an opportunity to practice preemptive nourishment. For example, if you're about to attend a three-hour meeting, eat something beforehand so you don't come out uncomfortably ravenous and shaky.

Full Moon Week

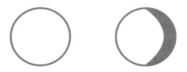

Includes Waning Gibbous

Element: Earth (skeletal, integumentary, and digestive systems)

Theme: Maintain momentum

The Full Moon initiates the waning half of the lunar cycle. In my early astrology days, I was so confused about the Full Moon's association with Earth. It felt fiery to me. But its job is to uncover the bones, or Earth, of things. The Full Moon is the truth teller of the phases, shining brightly on everything we've created, exposing whether or not it's what we intended. As the word *full* implies, under the Full Moon, life is full, and sometimes we can feel overwhelmed. To stay comfortable, after its swift peak, it's wise to move into a time of pruning.

This might look like saying no more often or putting fewer things on the to-do list. Yes, you may have your greatest energetic capacity under the Full Moon, but this energy is only sustained if it's used on the things that matter. It's easy to fritter away Full Moon energy and have nothing but exhaustion to show for it. The Full Moon is associated with the harvest, and its purpose is not to do more but to store more energy for the waning weeks ahead.

FULL MOON MOVEMENT

Aim to feel: Sustained

The Full Moon is the climax of the cycle, and the days and hours immediately surrounding it can feel supercharged. Working near, or even pushing slightly beyond your personal exercise threshold may feel aligned and exciting. Pro tip: This may shift depending on the zodiac sign in which the Full Moon occurs. But the greater lesson of the Full Moon is sustainability. Once the Full Moon is past, swiftly transition your intention from intensity to endurance. Whatever growth you experienced during the waxing half of the cycle, you want to maintain and carry with you into the next one. Integrate your new strengths and skills but keep longevity in mind. Ensure that movement sustains your energy rather than steals from it.

A common complaint right after the Full Moon's peak is exhaustion and body pain or stiffness. This is what I call the Full Moon hangover or crash, and it might be a clue that you've overextended earlier in the cycle. If this is the case, increased high-intensity movement is *not* the best strategy. Please take some time off. If you still wish to exercise, do some active recovery, increase the length of your warm-ups and cooldowns, and opt for gentler movement that encourages emotional and physical circulation.

FULL MOON NUTRITION

Aim to feel: Satisfied

As I said before, the Full Moon is associated with the harvest and conjures images of bounty, community, and storing food for the seasons ahead. Under the Full Moon, connect with the pleasurable and celebratory aspects of eating. Focus on foods and feeding patterns that not only sustain you during this busy time, but leave you feeling satiated. Use the Full Moon phase as an opportunity to befriend the sensation of fullness. How does it feel to be satisfied and what foods and amount of food truly create this feeling for you? Don't be surprised if this reflection is uncomfortable at first. Many of us have been conditioned to feel guilty when we eat—or even think about—the foods we enjoy. Sadness, fatigue, feeling cold, joint pain, and overeating are all clues that your body may not feel completely supported during this time. Eating to uncomfortable fullness is a normal response to deprivation. If you experience this during the Full Moon, rather than feeling discouraged, consider where deprivation may have snuck in earlier in the cycle. When we restrict food and forbid satisfaction, even subtly, we trigger a primal fear in the body that we won't have enough for "winter," or when food might be scarce. Although it may feel counterintuitive and even frightening at first, experiencing satisfaction is a vital part of cultivating a free and healthy relationship with food.

Last Quarter Moon Week

Includes Waning Crescent

Element: Water (endocrine, immune, and lymphatic systems; emotions)

Theme: Pause and make space

The Last Quarter Moon is the halfway point between the Full Moon and the next New Moon. We're on our way to emptiness. This is a time of completion, but unlike its waxing counterpart, the Last Quarter phase doesn't complete by building or producing but by pausing. It's a formless and timeless space where we learn that slowing down is often the most efficient and productive thing we can do. If possible, create more breaks and flexibility in your schedule. The body's resources are beginning to wane, and you may notice a significant shift in energy as the week progresses. This is natural, even helpful, and some-thing to embrace. If we chronically resist the inward pivot of this phase, over time we may find ourselves consumed by an extended period of fatigue. The refreshing and quickening parts of the cycle never come, and instead we feel stuck in a waning experience. The Last Quarter phase teaches that we do not need to be full and bright all the time to get where we want to go.

LAST QUARTER MOON MOVEMENT

Aim to feel: Flexible

Moving toward darkness doesn't mean we must stop exercising. When done mindfully, movement supports the completion of a cycle by acting as a processor or outlet. Moving, sweating, and breathing allow us to release our burdens, express emotion, and even expel toxins through the skin and lungs. This is the Water phase of the lunar cycle, which beckons us to bring more fluidity and softness into our movement practice. You could incorporate more mobility, flexibility, or bodyweight work into your routine. Or focus on moving with grace, which can be done whether you're a dancer or a weightlifter. But regardless of how you choose to move, cultivating a flexible, self-accepting mindset is the most important Last Quarter lesson. Toward the end of this phase, you're not likely to perform with the same vigor and drive as you did in earlier weeks. Allow yourself to make any midsession adjustments as necessary to feel comfortable. If that means doing less (or more) than you planned, that's just fine. During some late waning cycles, your interest in movement may disappear altogether—let that be okay. Trust yourself.

LAST QUARTER MOON NUTRITION

Aim to feel: Nurtured

"Release" is a popular buzzword for all the waning phases, including the Last Quarter. Yes, the Moon is emptying out, but please don't confuse themes of "release" and "letting go" with food "cleanses" or "detoxes." I have nothing against religious fasts and food observances, and that's not what I'm speaking about here. But as lunar movement and nutrition become more popular, please beware the new age hyper-spiritualizing of deprivation, implying that limiting food intake during this phase makes one more virtuous or spiritual. Withholding nutrients from the body has nothing to do with virtue and nothing to do with the Last Quarter Moon.

Rather, when the Moon wanes, the focus pivots from the external world to the internal world. The Last Quarter Moon is an opportunity to "release" all external messages about food (yes, even those touted by influencers, experts, or gurus) and tune in to internal ones. Use this phase to develop your nourishment intuition, which involves the ability to perceive internal cues as they arise and then attend to them compassionately. You've been developing this skill all cycle, but because the Last Quarter phase is both quieting and associated with the body's subtle Water systems—including the hormones, lymph, and emotions—it can be easier to get in touch with your internal food guidance. If consciously slowing down is new to you, it's normal for physical or emotional discomfort to bubble up at first. Choose foods and feeding practices that reinforce your own voice and make you feel heard, safe, and resourced enough to attend to these things gently.

Syncing with Menses

Before touching on menses, I want to be clear that my work in astro-nutrition and astro-fitness, although it has some natural overlap with the menstrual cycle, isn't a menstrual cycle system. It's an astrological system for all bodies, regardless of sex or gender, that takes numerous cosmic and biological rhythms into account. However, how to sync this system with the menstrual cycle is one of the most frequent questions I receive. But the answer is extremely variable depending on the health and needs of the person I'm working with.

   If we roughly superimpose the menstrual and lunar cycles, menstruation matches up with the New Moon and ovulation with the Full Moon. But menstrual cycles come at many different times. Some people bleed with the Full Moon instead, or perhaps the Crescent or Quarter Moon. And because both cycles are slightly variable in length from month to month, your bleeding pattern may gradually change throughout the year. All of this is normal and okay. No matter when you bleed during the real-time lunar calendar, if your cycle is regular, your hormonal ebbs and flows still imitate the waxing and waning Moon.

   You have a choice. You can move and eat with the real-time lunar cycle or you can take this same pattern and line it up with your menstrual cycle. There's no wrong choice, but there may be a wiser choice depending on your current hormonal health. I do a mash-up. I prefer living in alignment with the real-time astrology for most of the month and making small adjustments at menses and ovulation as needed. I can afford to do this because my cycle is regular and my body is highly adapted to exercise. But if my hormonal health were to change, I'd make room for more significant menstrual cycle adjustments. There's always an exception, but if your cycle is irregular, meaning it doesn't come at normal intervals, or if you're postmenopausal, or on birth control and not having a period, I suggest aligning with the real-time Moon to mimic some healthy cyclicality.

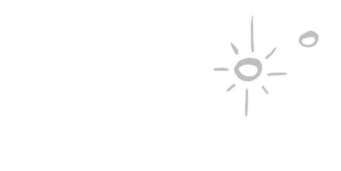

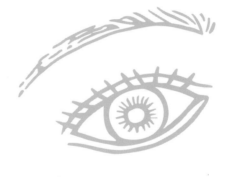

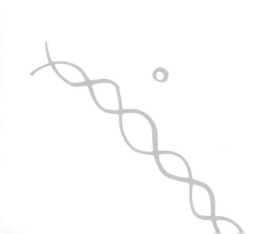

THE
SIGNS

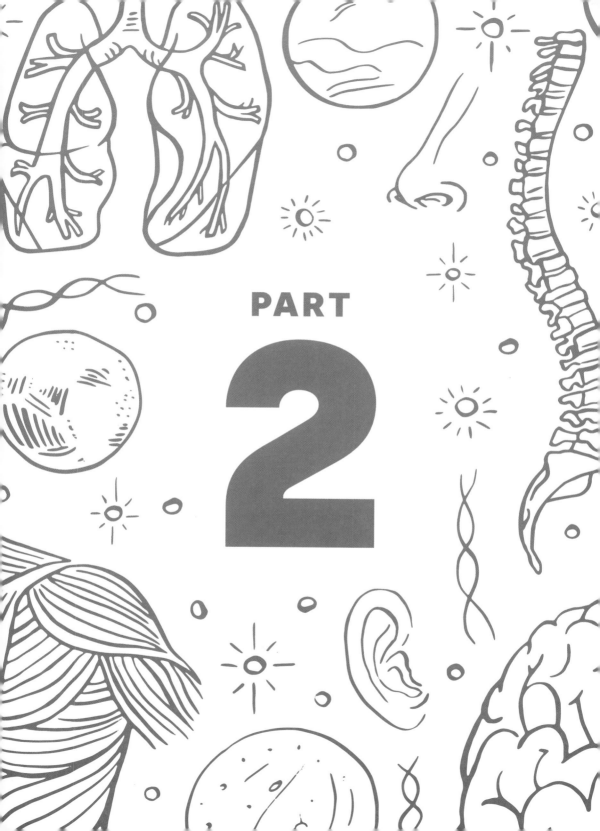

PART

2

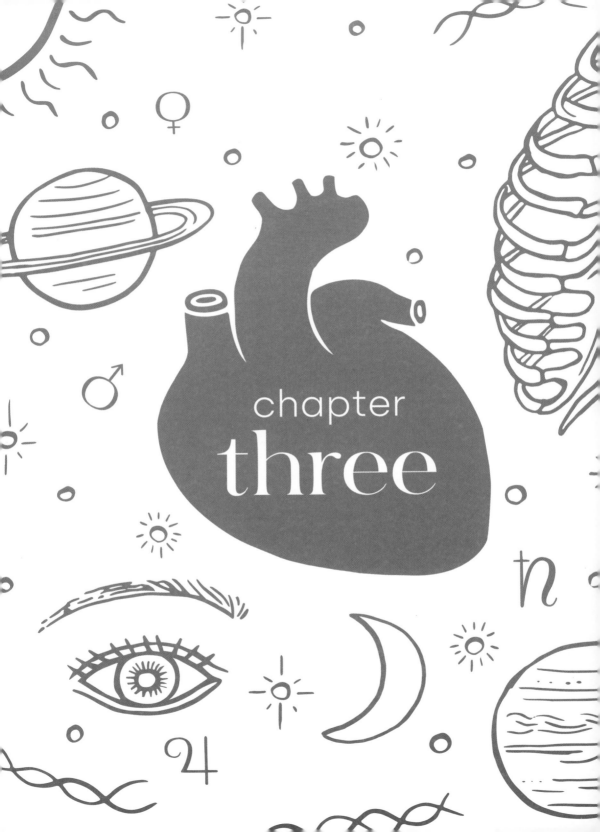

chapter
three

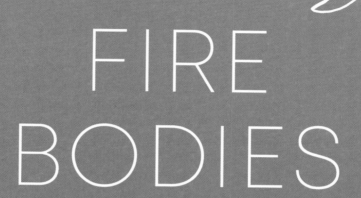

FIRE
BODIES

Signs: Aries, Leo, Sagittarius
Qualities: Hot, Dry

All the elements are essential to life, but Fire is our vitality. Its burning warms, animates, enlivens, and protects us. Fire is an agent of transformation, and that's what makes it so crucial. It cooks our food and initiates the many chemical reactions required to digest it—food into energy, energy into action, action into need, and so on. Fire both liberates and requires energy. It's the spark behind the brain, heart, muscle, metabolism, digestion, vision, and every chemical and enzymatic reaction in the body. Fire makes things go.

Fire is hot and dry, and it moves in an upward direction. These qualities give Fire its speed and precision. The Fire signs and planets are associated with organs and functions that pulse, blaze, and respond instantly and urgently. Healthy Fire reflects a healthy life force. We see this in an efficient pathogen-killing fever or in a lifesaving adrenaline surge. The dry quality gives Fire's body systems a very clear purpose and narrow margin of error. When they're off, it's painfully obvious and often dangerous.

People dominant in Fire run hotter. They may have naturally fast metabolisms, or they're so mentally and physically active that they simply require more fuel. Fire is action-oriented and feels most like itself when it's busy or creatively consumed. This element is mesmerizing; it captures our attention, and Fire people follow suit with their passion and enthusiasm. Fire must be fed to continue burning, and these people desire a steady diet of inspiration. Fire people are change agents, and their fervor paves a path for the future.

Fire bodies are naturally strong and robust, but as with all elements, great gifts can become roadblocks. When Fire flares out of control, we burn ourselves and others. Accidents, injuries, emergencies, rage, dehydration, and acidity are also aspects of Fire. And if Fire is untended, it burns out and all that remains is a pile of ash. Lifestyles that are too hot and too fast may prematurely snuff out Fire bodies or leave them with inflammatory conditions later in life. In Fire self-care, we want to make sure Fire always stays lit but never burns out of control. When Fire is contained and well fed, the body and mind are sharp, brilliant, and full of life.

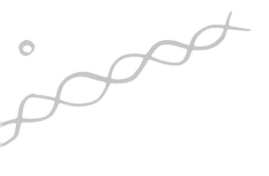

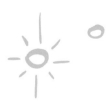

Supporting Fire Nutritionally

Astrology and the body are dynamic, and you can have too much, too little, or neutral Fire at any given time. Eating to support your Fire may look different throughout your life. Whether it's days, months, or years apart, you may find yourself cycling through periods of eating to decrease or increase Fire.

FIRE NUTRITION

Decreasing Fire	Increasing Fire
Cooling teas (chamomile, mint)	Alliums (chives, garlic, leeks, onions, shallots)
Copious water	Iron-rich animal protein (beef, chicken, turkey, sardines)
Fish	"Quick-burning" food, such as white rice and starchy vegetables
Fresh fruit and vegetables juices	
High-quality dairy	Plant iron sources (amaranth, beet greens, black-eyed peas, broccoli, chickpeas, collards, kale, lentils, molasses, pumpkin seeds, quinoa, spinach)
Lemon and lime	
Lightly steamed or raw food	
"Slow-burning" food, such as whole grains	Traditional blood-building foods (beets, deep-red foods, lamb, organ meats)
Water-rich fruits (apples, berries, melons, oranges, peaches, tomatoes)	Warming spices (black pepper, cardamom, cinnamon, cumin, curry, ginger, paprika, turmeric)
Water-rich vegetables (bell peppers, cabbage, celery, cucumbers, lettuce, mushrooms, zucchini)	Water with added minerals
	Well-cooked food and hot drinks

Foods and Practices That May Disturb Fire
Excess amounts of alcohol
Excess amounts of caffeine, especially in the form of energy drinks
Excess consumption of highly processed meats, such as bacon or sausage
Excess amounts of fried food
Hydrogenated oils, trans fats, and using any oil above its smoke point

ARIES

Aries Anatomy

Aries is often described as a headstrong leader and visionary, so it's no surprise that it rules the head, brain, and eyes. These parts of the body allow us not only to perceive the world but also to create it. Aries is a sign of action and so are its body systems. This sign's physical network is lightning fast, from brain impulses to the optic nerve to the adrenal glands' instant response to threat. There's almost no space between the impulse and the reaction, which makes this sign equal parts brilliant and daring.

Mode	Ruling Planet
Cardinal	Mars

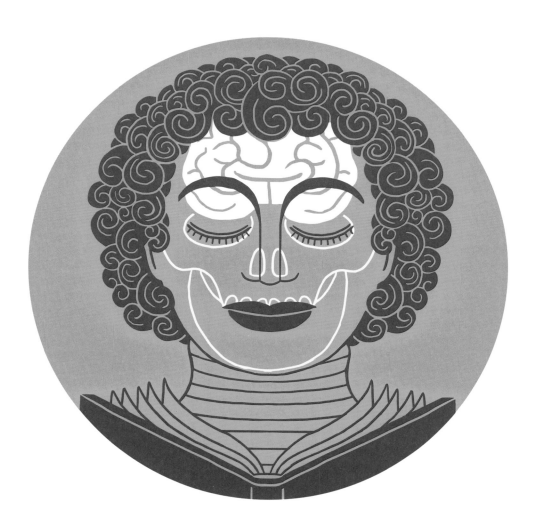

+ Head, including all bones and muscles of the skull and face

+ Brain

+ Cranial nerves

+ Eyes

+ Upper jaw

+ Upper teeth

+ Adrenal glands

Aries Nutrition

Gesture: Resilience

Aries energy is like lightning. It flashes quickly and dramatically and then disappears. This is exactly what you need in a survival situation, but in daily nutrition, you want to moderate Aries Fire so that its output is constant and sustainable. When imbalanced, it's common for the Aries body to act as though everything is an emergency. Supportive Aries nutrition communicates to the body that it's safe and doesn't need to call in the troops. The main ways to stabilize Aries nutritionally are to feed the brain, regulate blood sugar, and nourish the adrenal glands by developing stress resilience.

Aries is ruled by Mars, which means Mars-associated nutrients are typically nourishing for this sign. Mars rules acids of all kinds, including amino acids and fatty acids. Both are primary in supporting the brain and ensuring it operates smoothly. Instead of acting like a haphazard electrical storm, a healthy Aries brain strikes hot when it needs to and refrains when it doesn't. This is the balancing work of neurotransmitters. Aries disorders such as anxiety and epilepsy are linked to neurotransmitter imbalances. Amino acids are the building blocks of protein, but they're also used to synthesize neurotransmitters. Fatty acids are neuroprotective and grounding, and they regulate Aries Fire by keeping brain-cell membranes intact. Balanced Aries nutrition is full of healthy fats and high-protein foods that support proper neurotransmitter synthesis and function. Stock up on classic brain foods, including leafy greens, fatty fish, nuts, seeds, berries, organic ghee or butter, and eggs (be sure to eat the yolk), and try to eat protein at every meal. What type of protein you consume (animal or plant protein) is up to you and also may depend on whether your Fire is currently neutral, or in a state of excess or deficiency. If you're in a season of Fire excess, consuming a higher ratio of plant to animal protein may feel best, while the reverse may feel best during Fire deficiency. See the "Fire Nutrition" table at the beginning of the chapter for more info.

Before you run to try a high-fat diet with zero carbs, remember that Aries's nutritional priority is resilience and moderating stress—including physical stress. When we don't have the carbohydrates we need and our blood sugar levels rise or fall rapidly, our bodies are physically stressed. This triggers the body's emergency system, the adrenal glands, to kick into gear. Extreme dietary approaches, including the low-carb craze, typically backfire for this sign. Diets are not only mental stressors but also major physical stressors that trigger the Aries body to hyperrespond. Instead, begin relating to each macronutrient as a valuable player in your personal energy management. Carbohydrates offer a quick and accessible form of energy to the brain and body, while protein and fat create staying power and allow that energy to hang around longer. Unless Aries is dealing with a health imbalance, most of the time, getting all three macronutrients at meals is very stabilizing for blood sugar and will keep the body's stress response in check.

But eating carbs at night is bad, right? Wrong. This is a common nutrition myth. Let's reframe it. Blood sugar and cortisol have an inverse relationship. When blood sugar drops too low, the adrenal glands release cortisol to get those sugars back up. Increased cortisol at night means disrupted sleep and poor body repair (cortisol breaks down tissue). To encourage low cortisol in the evening, try eating a few more stabilizing carbs such as carrots, squash, potatoes, other starchy vegetables, beans, and whole grains.

Because Aries moves into high stress states so rapidly, it may not register hunger until it's uncomfortably ravenous, irritable, or has a headache. Stress can suppress the appetite, and over time, living in chronic stress can silence your body's hunger cues. If this is you, as you learn to moderate stress and get reacquainted with your hunger cues, make sure you have some snacks on hand that are fast and easy to grab. Don't expect to have the patience or brainpower to make supportive food choices or come up with an elaborate meal when you're already shaky with hunger. Eat a little something to regain composure and then approach cooking or picking up a fuller meal from a more grounded and comfortable place. Another planning tip is to know your busiest time of day and have a food strategy in place. If it's morning, pre-prepare breakfasts. If it's evening, always preplan dinner so you don't get stranded feeling uncomfortably hungry. You may also consider using fresh food delivery services, online grocery shopping, and precut or frozen vegetables, as well as filling your kitchen with appliances that cook quickly, such as an electric pressure cooker.

Separating Food and Stress

Although sometimes unavoidable, try to minimize gobbling food down in the car or at meetings. It's important for Aries to be diligent about separating food and stress so that the body doesn't correlate eating with "danger." Begin meals by placing your hands on your adrenal glands and taking three deep breaths. (Your adrenal glands are on top of your kidneys, above your low back and at the bottom of your rib cage on either side.) Thank them for all the work they do to protect you and let them know you're not in danger right now.

~~~~~~

Moderating Aries's stress may also include refraining from foods that create an inflammatory response in your body. Consuming foods that you're intolerant of or sensitive to increases physical stress and rings the adrenal alarm bell. Food reactions tend to be more obvious for Aries and may include sharp stomachache, migraine, headache, dizziness, or mood changes; subtler signals could be increased pulse rate or body temperature, sweating, or light sensitivity. Although Aries tends to love it, caffeine may be one such trigger. Caffeine creates what I think of as false Fire. It may feel like a boost in the moment, but instead of feeding Aries's Fire, caffeine creates a crash-and-burn effect, stressing the adrenal glands. Explore calming herbal teas, such as chamomile, peppermint, and lemon balm. Herbal coffee substitutes that include roots—dandelion, burdock, and chicory, for example—are also great choices. If, like me, you enjoy your morning coffee ritual, try to save it for after breakfast. At the very least, wait until you've had a large glass of water and pair your coffee with some fat.

On top of adding to stress, too much caffeine is also dehydrating. Although all the Fire signs can struggle with dehydration, Aries's connection to the adrenal glands makes water consumption and electrolyte balance especially important. Try to drink at least half your bodyweight in ounces of water per day. You may need to adjust this amount depending on climate and activity level. If you're chronically thirsty and fatigued and you don't have high blood pressure, try adding about ⅛ teaspoon of high-quality sea salt to a glass of water upon waking or making a homemade electrolyte drink (see below).

~~~~~~

Aries Electrolyte Drink

Store-bought electrolyte drinks often have a lot of artificial dyes, flavorings, and sweeteners. Instead, put all of the following ingredients in a jar or glass and mix them together for a healthy thirst quencher.

+ ½ cup water
+ ½ cup coconut water
+ Juice of ½ lemon
+ ⅛ teaspoon Himalayan pink salt
+ ½–1 teaspoon honey

~~~~~~

Aries Movement

Gesture: Peak

Aries doesn't typically have a lot of patience when it comes to working out. It loathes endurance and wants things to be sweaty and efficient. Movement quickly turns into competition, and if other people are around, Aries wants to finish first. As a cardinal sign, Aries initiates the characteristics of Fire, bringing flames out of thin air. This is spark energy, and in the world of athletics, this means Aries reaches peak performance in record time. Classic Aries workouts are extremely intense, short, and may leave you gasping on the floor. Sprinters, wrestlers, and professional athletes know this feeling well. For an Aries workout, the aim is to do as much work as possible in the shortest amount of time. This requires appropriate body prep and simple routines with a straightforward approach.

No matter if you're lifting, running, or doing a quick yoga flow, the warm-up may be the most important part of an Aries routine. When Aries is involved, it's tempting to skip this and go straight into the main work for the day. You may think this is saving time, but it's majorly reducing your workout's effectiveness. If you go straight into hard work without appropriately prepping the nervous system, the body is going to use the workout as a warm-up and be more vulnerable to injury (a common Aries issue). Simply put—you can go through the motions, but you just can't work at your personal peak with a cold body and a sleepy nervous system. A good warm-up should leave you slightly damp and with audible breath.

Head to clairegallagher.co/bodyastro for video examples of Aries movements.

Aries workouts can easily become purposeless sweat fests, which may feel good in the moment but get you nowhere long term. To use Aries energy effectively, you must understand intensity. There's perceived intensity and actual intensity—how hard you *feel* you're working versus how hard you're actually working. For Aries workouts to be effective, you want to reach actual intensity occasionally, instead of perceived intensity daily. Let's pretend you go to a high-intensity boot camp class every day and this plan goes pretty well until later in the week when the excess strain begins to add up. You're tired, sore, and uninterested in your workout, but you're determined to do it anyway. Because you've come to class prefatigued, you won't be able to reach your personal peak. Yes, it's going to *feel* extremely hard (perceived intensity) because you've worn yourself out over the week, but it's not actually hard—meaning your body can't work at its highest capacity. It's not refreshed enough to even mount the proper physiological response. This is a waste of your time and resources.

To keep Aries movement effective, you need to use intensity intelligently and, honestly, sparingly. Long term, this means making sure your program is well rounded and that you're not trying to do high-intensity exercise every day of the week. Reaching actual peak intensity one to two times per week for just a few minutes is plenty. More than that tends to create a negative hormonal cascade.

Breath of Fire

As the name implies, Breath of Fire is very invigorating and brings a lot of energy and oxygen to the Aries-ruled head and brain. I might use Breath of Fire on a long drive (eyes open!) or during an afternoon slump for a pick-me-up. It's also expulsive and cleansing, and it may help you shake off some physical or emotional stress. I don't recommend Breath of Fire before bed.

Sit comfortably with a tall spine and gently place your hands on your belly. Take a big inhale through your nose. Exhale rapidly and sharply through your nose while contracting your abdomen. Release your belly as you inhale. The nasal inhale is quick but should feel natural and reflexive. Repeat. This is a rapid breath, so go at your own pace and start small—even ten breaths is very powerful. As you get comfortable, increase your speed and work up to a round of fifty. Finish with a long inhale and exhale.

Aries Strength and Conditioning

For Aries strength and conditioning, keep things hot and efficient with some no-nonsense strength work. There are many ways to do this, but one of my favorites is on-the-minute training (often shortened to EMOM for "every minute on the minute"). For example, ten barbell back squats every minute on the minute for five to ten minutes is some fiery strength work.

When it comes to conditioning, Aries challenges us to leave it all out on the floor. One way to do this is with a short circuit of exercises (less than five) that you perform as fast as possible. To keep intensity high, choose straightforward exercises that allow you to focus on speed, such as simple variations of squats, deadlifts, kettlebell swings, overhead presses, and maybe some running or jump rope. When you finish, rest long enough to where you can repeat the circuit again at an equal or higher intensity. If you're truly working at a high level, you'll need way more than ten seconds to refresh—we're talking anywhere from one to five minutes.

Aries Running

Nothing mirrors Aries energy more perfectly than a sprint. Although there are all kinds of sprint durations, Aries wants to focus on maximum effort, which means setting a pace you can only hold for ten to twenty seconds at the most. Choose flat terrain or a track to keep speed as high as possible. Fully recover between sprints so that you can hit this intensity again and again. Bring in some Aries competition and grab a friend to race against, or race against yourself and try to beat your fastest time.

Alternatively, you could use a Tabata format. Set an interval timer for eight intervals of twenty seconds of work and ten seconds of rest (four minutes total). Run as hard as you can during the twenty-second work periods.

Aries Yoga

Aries energy is most readily reflected in vigorous forms of vinyasa yoga such as ashtanga, which is fast paced and physically demanding. Power yoga and fusion classes that incorporate cardio intervals are right up Aries's alley too. Working on your headstand would definitely be an Aries thing to do. But you can also emulate Aries in restorative practices that focus on relaxing the Aries body areas, including the eyes, head, and face. Don't forget breathing practices as well—Breath of Fire (see sidebar) definitely fits the Aries criteria.

Other Aries Sports and Classes

+ Boot camp classes

+ CrossFit

+ Extreme adventure sports that create an adrenaline rush (especially in fiery, hot environments)

+ Fire hooping and other activities that use real flames

+ HIIT (high intensity interval training) classes

+ Military and tactical training

+ Mixed martial arts and other combat sports

+ Races, competitions, and sporting events of all kinds

Aries Conditions

Aries is a very robust sign, and its illnesses tend to be just as robust. The good news is that if Aries is healthy, it tends to get sick very quickly and recover just as quickly. Aries imbalances mimic the urgent warrior energy of Mars and may come on fervently and suddenly and could occur as an event or accident. These conditions are typically acute and extreme in expression; they aren't easily ignored. Because Aries rules the head, these imbalances tend to flare upward, but they're often mirroring a much wider network of inflammation in the rest of the body and lifestyle. Aries conditions may present in the following ways:

Accident proneness

Acne or rash on head, neck, or face

Addison's disease, Cushing's syndrome, and other diseases of the adrenal glands

Adrenal dysfunction and cortisol imbalances

Anaphylaxis

Anger and irritability

Anxiety and panic attacks

Cerebrovascular events and diseases

Chronic stress

Dehydration

Fever

Headache and migraine

Insomnia

Mental illness

Neurological disorders, including Alzheimer's, Bell's palsy, epilepsy, and hundreds of others

Traumatic brain injury and concussion

Vision problems, eye strain, eye pain, eye injury, and eye infection

Aries is great in a crisis, but if it's creating crisis to avoid something else or to stay energized and alert, Aries may need to make some adjustments. Imbalanced Aries may feel anxious, depressed, or frustrated when it's not rushing around at school or work and may avoid these feelings by keeping extra busy. In the gym, Aries may feel like it's giving maximum effort and receiving minimum benefit. And in relationships, it may initiate tension just to give its Fire something to feed on. There's nothing wrong with being a go-getter, but Aries tends to rely on the body's emergency system rather than truly learning how to manage stress. If this goes on for too long and the emergency state becomes a daily experience, a classic Aries crash-and-burn is imminent. At the lowest point of this crash, Aries may feel completely disconnected from its natural passion, drive, and interest.

Aries, a powerhouse, can go a long time ignoring the whispers of burn-out. This is severely complicated by the fact that a high-stress lifestyle is applauded by modern society. But sooner or later, physiological corners are cut to keep the body functioning at the high level that Aries demands. Maybe it just starts with a few headaches, being wired instead of tired, or feeling more irritable than usual. But the tricky thing about Aries is that once its work, creative, or athletic performance begins to dwindle, rather than stepping back and asking what the body needs, its default is to push harder, which only ends up driving the stress cycle deeper. Some may even take on extra work or use extreme dieting and excess amounts of high-intensity exercise for short-lived shots of cortisol and endorphins. Living in a chronic state of emergency rapidly burns up the body's resources. Soon, basic body repair and detoxification, as well as digestive and reproductive health, go out the window because they aren't considered essential in times of high alert. In extreme cases, this is when acute and more serious illness may pop up and stop Aries in its tracks.

To get back to true power, Aries must completely step out of this cycle. It's counterintuitive that doing less will allow Aries to do more, but that's exactly how this sign works. This is just like the inflammatory process in the body. A balanced inflammatory response is quick to act, initiating the healing process and then settling down. But when we're exhausted, the inflammatory response becomes inefficient; it lingers and may never complete its work. This is when the chronic inflammation so common for this sign begins to take root. Similarly, when Aries Fire is healthy, it's efficient—it gets the job done and then comes back to baseline to refuel, allowing it to show up in power again and again and again.

Other Planets in Aries
Mercury in Aries

Mercury in Aries is a rapid responder and may make for a brilliant mind. But if overworked, the brain may feel like it's on fire, too quick to catch, or responding before information has been fully processed. The nutritional focus is to stabilize and even slow nervous system function. This Mercury needs large amounts of protein and healthy fat to keep it feeling steady. Caffeine isn't recommended.

Typically this Mercury likes to move fast, but it tires quickly and bores easily. If well placed, it's speedy and coordinated, but it can become clumsy and injury prone if overtaxed. Exercise needs to be stress relieving instead of stress inducing, meaning high-intensity exercise should be used and scheduled with care. This Mercury needs a vigorous stress outlet, such as sprints or boxing, but too much can backfire and create more stress. Instead of forcing this impatient Mercury to endure lengthy workouts or slowing and confusing it with complex movements and routines, it's best to keep workouts simple and efficient.

Venus in Aries

For Venus in Aries, negative food reactions may manifest as facial acne, headaches, congestion, nerve pain, or dental issues. The connection between adrenal function and sex hormone production is primary and, if overwhelmed, this Venus may experience hormonal imbalances. Eating for hormonal and adrenal health is a priority, and for Venus in Aries, this approach typically involves the use of therapeutic oils and fatty acids.

This Venus knows what it wants and it wants it now. There's often a lot of pressure to immediately see exercise "results," whether aesthetic or performance based. Quick fixes, crash exercising, and dieting may be attractive, but they will just get this Venus further away from what it truly desires. These things may exacerbate cortisol imbalances, which can eat away at lean muscle mass.

Mars in Aries

Mars in Aries is a fast metabolizer and may need more calories or more frequent meals. Mars-ruled nutrients such as protein and iron are used rapidly, and simple carbohydrates may be necessary in appropriate amounts at the right time. This Mars doesn't have much patience when it comes to food planning, shopping, and prepping. Take advantage of meal-planning apps or grocery shopping services, and focus on simple meals that don't take too long to prepare. Always have high-protein snacks and water on hand. Negative food reactions are often acute and intense.

This is a very competitive and often naturally athletic Mars. This Mars is motivated by urgency, being the best, or finishing first. It will also thrive in preparing for competitive events or simply structuring workouts as challenges, races, or competitions. Try competing against the clock, previous personal records, or another fiery friend. Although often unnatural, try to keep movement longevity in mind. It's easy for this Mars to use up all its Fire early in life, collecting quite a few injuries along the way. Moderate your output so that you can enjoy movement throughout your entire life.

Jupiter in Aries

Jupiter in Aries is very enthusiastic and prone to acidity and overheating. This Jupiter may show symptoms of a "hot" liver and experience lots of blood and energy rushing to the head. This could manifest as hot flashes, excessive brain activity, high blood pressure, migraines, irritability, insomnia, and other indications of excess flaring Fire. It may be helpful for this Jupiter to regularly consume energetically cooling foods, such as vegetable juices and raw foods. Symptoms may be aggravated by heat in the form of excess stress or alcohol or fried, greasy, and spicy foods.

When starting an exercise program, this Jupiter may be excited at first but soon lose interest or get distracted by the next exciting thing that comes along. It's always seeking that initial spark of inspiration. Work with this natural impulse as you create an exercise routine. Give yourself lots of movement variety and excitement while still having an overarching plan or direction.

Saturn in Aries

Saturn in Aries may struggle with getting enough blood and oxygen to the brain, often resulting in poor cognition and coordination, headaches, and fatigue. To offset this condition, this Saturn can prioritize foods, herbs, and spices that encourage circulation—try cinnamon, garlic, ginger, onion, or turmeric. Saturn often indicates areas of nutritional deficiency, and when in Aries it's common to need more protein, iron, B vitamins, and amino acids.

This Saturn may find it hard to reach high-intensity states in exercise or may struggle with athletic burnout more frequently than other planets in this sign. It's important to ensure that your workout program adds to your energy level instead of subtracts from it. Any fatigue, chronic injury, or lack of motivation is often rooted in this Saturn's struggle with blood and oxygen circulation. If you're in a season of fatigue or recovery, make global blood flow your exercise priority instead of high intensity. Apart from regular workouts, incorporate bursts of movement or inversions throughout the workday to keep yourself alert.

Uranus in Aries

Like Mercury in Aries, Uranus in Aries needs a stabilizing nutritional approach that calms the nervous system. Sharp headaches and other hot, acute conditions in the brain, mood, and face are possible. This Uranus has an affinity for fast and furious movement but may be accident prone.

Neptune in Aries

For Neptune in Aries, poor digestive health may manifest as cognitive fog, sinus congestion, somnolence, and fatigue. Like Venus in Aries, this Neptune often needs targeted adrenal nourishment and may need to use titrated exercise as a gentle stimulant.

Aries Nourishment Checklist	Aries Movement Checklist
Gesture: Resilience	**Gesture:** Peak
✦ Carry snacks and water	✦ Competition against self or others
✦ Hydrate	✦ Effective warm-up
✦ Moderate caffeine	✦ Efficient and straightforward
✦ Plan ahead	✦ Intelligent use of intensity
✦ Prioritize protein	✦ Quick bursts at maximum effort
✦ Slow down to eat	✦ Short duration

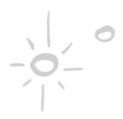

LEO

Leo Anatomy

Leo rules the Sun of the body—the heart. Nothing can exist without this vital orb or organ, and Leo's radiance, generosity, and desire to shine keep us alive. All of Leo's body areas circulate vitality. The heart and its vessels bring blood to every cell, while the spinal cord and myelin sheaths allow life-sustaining impulses to travel like omnidirectional rays. The Sun is our most proud and loyal light and, unlike the Moon, rises whole every day. Leo's anatomy reflects this integrity and consistency not only in the heart but also in the constant muscular support and uprightness of the spine.

Mode	Ruling Planet
Fixed	Sun

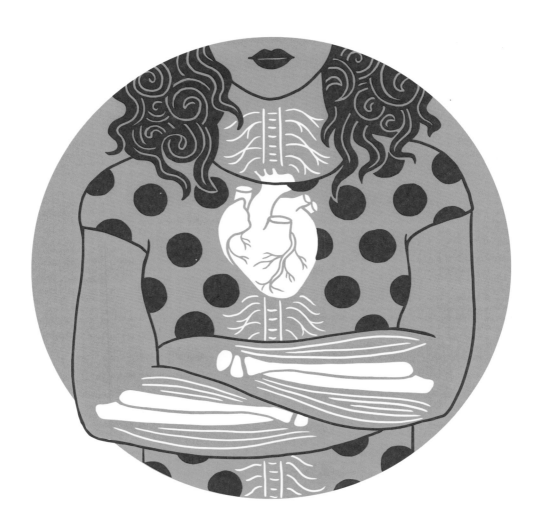

+ Heart

+ Aorta

+ Vena cava

+ Arterial system (with Sagittarius)

+ Muscles of the back (all, but especially the mid-back)

+ Spinal cord

+ Myelin sheaths of the nerves

+ Thoracic vertebrae

+ Radius, ulna, wrists, and muscles of forearms (with Gemini)

Leo Nutrition

Gesture: Heart(h) Food

When I learned that my Granny was a double Leo, this sign's food habits began to make perfect sense. Being well endowed with Leo myself, my fondest memories of Granny are her lavish family meals. I'm talking over-the-top extravagant: two main dishes, about six side dishes, and multiple desserts, all homegrown and made from scratch. At Thanksgiving, Granny would make a separate pumpkin pie just for me, and I could have unlimited fried eggs at breakfast, so long as I didn't tell Dad. Saturated fat was abundant and welcome—and this was back in the early nineties when we still thought it caused heart disease. Every Leo is a showboat, but not in the stereotypical way you might think. Granny certainly wasn't an extrovert, but that dinner table was her stage. For Leo, food is often a magnetizing, centripetal force meant to gather everything it loves together. It's the hearth of the zodiac.

Heart food, both physical and emotional, is the foundation of Leo nutrition. Eating for cardiovascular health is a hotly debated topic. Older astrological texts typically say that Leo should never eat meat or anything remotely fattening. But as we deepen our nutritional knowledge, we're watching the correlation between fat and heart disease shift. Does this mean that traditional astrological nutrition was wrong in this case? No. We just need to look at it a little differently.

It's true that meat and fat, especially animal fat, are energetically heating. It's also true that Leo is one of the hottest signs in the zodiac, and piling on more heat doesn't make much sense. Regardless of the season outside your window, ideal Leo nutrition mimics the height of summer. It's plentiful, fun, eye-pleasing, and mostly vegetables and fruit. A Leo plate is colorful and full of red, yellow, and orange foods—the colors of Leo's ruler, the Sun—and green foods, as green represents the energy center of the heart. It's natural for summer fare to be a little lighter and more cooling. So, treating meat as a condiment may work well for Leo. This might look like enjoying well-sourced animal protein once per day and allowing other protein sources such as beans and legumes to be the stars of the show sometimes. It could mean focusing on lighter proteins such as chicken, fish, or turkey, or simply ensuring your serving of meat is the size of your palm and the bulk of your meal comes from plants. Fully vegetarian approaches work well too, if healthy plant fats and oils—such as avocado, olive, coconut, nuts, and seeds—are a major part of the menu. Sometimes Leo is attracted to raw food because it's energetically cooling, but depending on the rest of your chart, too much of it could be aggravating for your digestion. I'm looking at you Leo and Water or Virgo combos. Instead, experiment with salads and dishes that have a combo of cooked and raw elements.

Royal Toppings

Fill your pantry with antioxidant sprinkles to quickly transform any meal into a Leo-worthy banquet: acai, black sesame seeds, blueberries, cacao nibs, flaxseed meal, goji berries, grape tomatoes, matcha powder, nori granules, pomegranate seeds, pistachios, sliced almonds, unsweetened shredded coconut, walnut pieces, and so on.

Leo's natural inclination toward rich food and generous spreads is this sign's inner food wisdom popping up. To feel satisfied, Leo needs a touch of daily decadence. Real butter, creamy sauces, dressings, and animal fat have a place on Leo's plate if it chooses. But Leo can also create this fit-for-royalty effect in other ways. Not every Leo meal needs to be elaborate, but if you're feeling inspired, use edible flower petals, dried lavender buds, citrus zest, and other decorative touches for a little dramatic flair. These delightful toppings not only satisfy Leo's visual appetite but also offer a ton of Fire-supporting nutrients.

Most Leo imbalances occur when the body's Fire doesn't circulate properly. Leo is prone to physical or emotional heart blockages as energy coagulates in the chest. Although heart disease is certainly one manifestation of this, consider others, such as fainting or depression. Regardless, when Fire is stuck, it burns and creates cellular damage in one area while the rest of the body is starved of heat and nutrients. Balanced Leo nutrition accounts for this by incorporating foods that relax the heart muscle; repair cellular damage; and move blood, heat, and nourishment throughout the body. Lots of fiber, antioxidant foods, and iron-rich vegetables fit the bill. Additionally, magnesium may be Leo's most important nutrient. Magnesium does hundreds of things, but in the realm of Leo, it regulates contractions in every muscle of the body, including the heart and the smooth muscle of the blood vessels. Increased dietary magnesium from almonds, avocados, dark leafy greens, pumpkin seeds, and even dark chocolate can open the door of the heart and help Leo Fire circulate more comfortably. But opening the heart doesn't just hinge on what we're eating but also how we're eating. Leo is nourished by connection. Even if you're dining solo, dedicate one meal per day as a time for self-celebration and heart connection. Leo is also nourished by the Sun. Try taking your meals in as much natural light as possible, or better yet, eat outside when you can.

~~~~~~~~~~~~~~~~~~~~~~~~

Heart-Centered Eating

Begin meals by placing one or both hands on your heart and checking in. What does this space feel like? Does your heart have enough room? Breathe into the area behind your heart and imagine it expanding the back of your body. If you experience physical or emotional congestion in your chest or abdomen while eating, try putting a bolster, cushion, or even a tennis ball against your thoracic spine, ideally right below your shoulder blades. This will force you to open your chest and create more room in your Leo body areas.

~~~~~~~~~~~~~~~~~~~~~~~~

Leo Movement

Gesture: Heart Tending

Just like nutrition, Leo movement hinges on physical and spiritual heart health. Cardiovascular exercise is a major part of this sign's fitness formula, but whether Leo likes cardio or not is debatable. Regardless, there tends to be a strong opinion about exercise that raises your heart rate—whether it's love, hatred, need, or obsession. But equally important is cultivating joy and contentment and using movement as a tool for healing and steadying the energetic heart.

Leo's health is highly attuned to solar cycles, and when we're working with the heart, we're symbolically working with the Sun. The Sun is a constant, dependable light whose variations are much simpler than the mysterious, quick-changing moods of the Moon. The Sun rises whole and complete every day and, like the Sun, healthy Leo reflects this by retaining its brightness, confidence, and magnetism no matter the external circumstances. Begin to think of cardiovascular exercise as building your own sunrise muscle—the ability to rise in full joy, contentment, and worth daily, regardless of your surroundings. Because it reflects the Sun's consistency, cyclical cardio is a Leo workout

Head to clairegallagher.co/bodyastro for video examples of Leo movements.

staple. Examples are cycling, jump rope, rowing, running, walking, or any other repetitive churning of the body. This type of rote movement is nourishing for fixed signs and has a place in their program, so long as it's used with intent. Cyclical cardio is great for increasing general fitness. It's also wonderful for creating global blood flow, which means it circulates nourishing and healing substances around the body, making it a valuable part of recovery. Plus, it simply makes us feel good and can be a reliable mood booster. But if cyclical movement is all we rely on, we aren't going to build a strong, multidimensional, and adaptable body.

Although it may sound counterintuitive, to cultivate solar steadiness we need to put the physical heart through highly unsteady conditions. Life is dynamic, and a happy heart is variable and adaptable. A quick, single-speed jog around the neighborhood won't get us there, but neither will a constant demand for the heart to work at its threshold. As a fixed sign, Leo tends to get locked into one type or one speed of exercise. Rather than enhancing Leo's natural qualities, this aggravates and exaggerates them, leading Leo toward inflammatory physical and mental states and overuse injuries.

Whether you like to get your cardio at the dance studio or the weight room, Leo thrives on a combined cardio approach that uses both sustainable and unsustainable paces. Sustainable work is slower and can be done for many minutes at a time. Unsustainable work is often referred to as the anaerobic threshold, where you're struggling to breathe. This all-out effort can only be sustained for a few minutes at the most. Right below threshold, where the line between sustainable and unsustainable begins to blur, is another important mode. This is where the most growth tends to happen for Leo because it teaches you how to control your effort and sustain a challenging pace without moving into exhaustion.

Leo Strength and Conditioning

As you know by now, Leo rules the back. To keep Leo nourished and injury-free in slower and heavier strength work, Leo's strength and conditioning program often needs to focus on the back of the body twice as much as it focuses on the front. During your training week, do twice as many pulling and hinging exercises—deadlifts, rows, kettlebell swings, and pull-ups, for example—than pushing exercises, such as bench presses and push-ups. Pulling exercises also help open the chest and heart, something Leo should always be mindful of. For a well-rounded Leo routine, finish up with back and spine mobility.

Ideal Leo conditioning is mixed modal, meaning it uses a combination of weighted, unweighted, and cyclical movements in the same workout. As someone with both natal Mars and Mercury in Leo, this is my favorite type of training. Not only is the mixed approach more interesting, but it also breaks up the training week and keeps us from the repetitive injuries often found in solely cyclical approaches. Because weight is involved, this style conditions the heart and builds strength endurance. To start, create a circuit with a cyclical movement, one or more weighted movements, and a bodyweight movement. Remember, you want to work with sustainable and unsustainable paces, and you can do this with just a few tweaks to routine format and intention. For sustainable work, your goal is to pace yourself. This will require intentional rest periods. For unsustainable work, throw pacing out the window and try to work at your personal threshold.

Pro tip: Unsustainable work is best saved for late First Quarter Moon week and right around the Full Moon, while sustainable work is a good choice during the late waning Moon and New Moon weeks (see chapter 2 for more lunar-cycle movement guidance).

Leo Running

Remember that Leo is a fixed Fire sign, which means it tends to like consistent movement such as cyclical, steady-state cardio. A thirty-minute jog at a moderate pace that you can sustain for an hour or more is a perfect example. But to keep Leo growing and balanced, challenge the heart with varying speeds and intensities. A tempo run is one of my favorite Leo tools because it teaches Leo how to increase its pace without burning out. There are endless tempo-run variations, but I like Leo's to take the form of a sandwich. Moderate effort is the bread on either side and threshold effort (right below race pace, where you can only speak a word or two) is the filling. I love this structure because the heart doesn't get to stop right after the challenge; it must adapt, come back down to moderate effort, and keep moving. The duration of each section is up to your needs and running experience, but for this sign I suggest keeping them equal.

Also, keep that Leo one-track stubbornness in check and make sure you're doing adequate cross-training. Picking up a yoga or strength-training class for runners even just a few times per month can keep you running a lot longer and happier.

Leo Yoga

Like the other Fire signs, Leo tends to be attracted to more vigorous yoga practice styles that create heat in the body. This can be done with flow speed, posture choice, breath (try just breathing through your nose), or room temperature. You'll often find Leo dripping with sweat in hot yoga classes. Leo, already really hot, may get aggravated if it does hot yoga every day, but when done in moderation, it's a wonderful Fire mover for this sign. (Leo energy tends to get stuck and needs help moving things out of the body—sweat is one such vehicle.) Hot room or not, a flow heavy on the Sun Salutations (*surya namaskar*) definitely hits the Leo spot. A great Leo flow also focuses on its body rulerships. Incorporate backbends, spinal twists, chest openers, and postures that open and support the mid back, right behind the heart. Some lesser-known Leo ruled body parts are the wrists and forearms. Strengthen these and get the heart pumping by working on your plank endurance and yoga push-ups (*chaturanga dandasana*).

Other Leo Sports and Classes

+ Any movement that brings you joy

+ Being the team captain or leader of any sport

+ Celebrity trainer methods

+ Cyclical cardio of all kinds (cycling, jump rope, rowing, running, walking)

+ Cheerleading

+ Circuit-training classes

+ Heart rate–based interval classes, such as Orangetheory

+ Sports with a performative element (competitive bodybuilding, dance, games, and matches)

Leo Conditions

Leo imbalances occur when the body's vitality doesn't circulate properly. All fixed signs are prone to getting stuck, but when the Sun of the body is blocked, things can get serious very quickly. When the heart is temporarily clouded over and its light is too weak, Leo may feel depressed, cold, or faint. But when the heart's heat is impeded for many years, we may see the buildup, stuck Fire, and inflammation of heart disease. Either way, the warmth of the heart is inconsistent, and when its light finally breaks through, we often see theatrical physical or emotional displays. Leo conditions may manifest as:

- Back pain
- Chest tightness, pain, or discomfort
- Circulatory issues
- Dehydration
- Demyelination and neurodegeneration
- Depression
- Heart disease
- Heart palpitations
- Heat rash, sunburn, skin cancer
- Heatstroke
- High cholesterol
- Postural issues, scoliosis
- Seasonal affective disorder
- Spinal cord injury, compression, or infection
- Spinal misalignments
- Syncope
- Tachycardia
- Vitamin D deficiency

The biggest hint that Leo may need to reframe its relationship to food and movement is when it begins approaching these things from a false sense of self. Beyond vitality, the Sun represents our identity. Because Leo is ruled by the Sun, distorted senses of self and pain around purpose and meaning frequently pop up as growth opportunities and weave their way into Leo's wellness approach. When Leo is harmonized, it reflects the Sun's benefic qualities. Its warm and generous light shines on all of us. Leo's self-assurance and confidence aren't turnoffs but inspiration for others to feel similarly about themselves. Leo is magnetizing without being demanding.

When Leo's inner light becomes harsh and blinding, we often see inflated senses of self. Leo's insecurity forces it to turn up the brightness, and there might be dramatic fits, pathological pride, and fixation with being the best, the brightest, the strongest, the most beautiful—fill in the blank. In food and movement, this behavior tends to coincide with an all-or-nothing mentality or an overly zealous devotion to a certain practice. Leo may take a self-righteous stance, believing its way of eating and exercising is superior and should work for everyone. This could also manifest as a strong-willed attachment to a protocol that's clearly not working for Leo or actively causing it harm. Leo may be too prideful to stop or simply blind to the damage. In fitness, this often shows up as cardio addiction or self-acceptance hinging on whether it did its workout or not. This is where the disease process in Leo begins, not in the protocol itself but in the gripping and often arrogant attachment to the approach.

When Leo's inner light is clouded over, we see deflated senses of self. This isn't better or worse than an inflated sense of self. It's equally inaccurate and rooted in insecurity. When the light is diminished, Leo will abandon itself and look elsewhere for brightness. Identity and meaning often hinge on another person or an audience and whether Leo feels needed, approved of, or desired. When Leo is in this state, self-care is rarely for the self. It's usually for another or perhaps to keep up appearances. If this Leo suffers rejection or loss, preparing a nourishing meal or exercising may feel purposeless because there's no one to do it for. Both distortions of self occur when Leo stops being self-generating and looks to others to generate its light instead.

Other Planets in Leo
Mercury in Leo

Mercury in Leo is creative and engaging, but its mood and cognitive ability are very sensitive to solar seasons. The nutrients of the Sun, especially vitamin D and magnesium, are especially necessary, and it may also need the support of light therapy. This idealistic Mercury can be very attached and loyal to dietary ideals long after they've stopped being productive.

This Mercury is prone to dehydration-related muscle spasms, as well as nerve pain in the wrists and forearms that is often rooted in the thoracic spine. It has a naturally high cardiovascular capacity but is prone to overdoing it and may commonly experience heart palpitations or flutters.

Venus in Leo

Venus in Leo loves extravagant displays and generous feasts but is equally concerned about its attractiveness. If it feels threatened, unappreciated, or unseen, the Leo Venus may turn to disordered eating or exercising to create a false sense of self-worth or value. Sometimes this Venus can feel weak and may need extra Fire-generating nutrients such as iron, protein, or B vitamins to bolster its heart force.

This Venus is drawn to movement modalities that are fun, flashy, and have a performative element, whether it's more creative or competitive. Again, the caution is becoming overly preoccupied with working out to look a certain way. This Venus may feel lightheaded or dizzy with extreme exertion and should pay attention to pre-workout fueling and electrolyte intake.

Mars in Leo

Mars in Leo is extra hot and may need to rely on a personalized anti-inflammatory menu occasionally. It can be aggravated by large amounts of alcohol, coffee, garlic, onions, spices, and other foods that are energetically hot and stimulating. It rapidly burns through iron, protein, and B vitamins and should be careful to get adequate amounts.

This Mars is motivated by passion and needs movement to be heart-full and inspiring. If it's inactive, it may experience restlessness, depression, or even high blood pressure or heart issues later in life. It loves the rush of intensity and may push itself to depletion or injury, especially in the back. This zealous Mars needs to ensure it has enough variation in its approach and isn't fixated only on high-intensity states.

Jupiter in Leo

Jupiter in Leo has a soft spot for richness. Allowing enjoyment and reconnecting with the pleasures of eating are health-protective behaviors. Jupiter in Leo can also accumulate a lot of heat. Depending on the rest of the chart, this Jupiter may occasionally need more cooling or even raw plant food as compared to other Leo placements.

Depending on the house placement, this Jupiter either feels very expanded and encouraged by exercise or totally uninterested and would rather get its fun elsewhere. Regardless, this placement needs an inspiring mixture of aerobic and anaerobic exercise to ensure long-term cardiovascular health. Healthy competition or a good cause might get this Jupiter moving.

Saturn in Leo

Saturn in Leo can experience constriction in both the heart and back. Opening the chest and watching posture during meals can be very therapeutic. Gentle walking after meals is also encouraged. This Saturn may be shy to admit it, but it needs nourishing affirmation and creativity like any other Leo planet. Use meals as conscious opportunities to bring warmth and lighthearted connection to your day.

This Saturn may either feel very averse to cardiovascular exercise or may prefer cyclical modalities over short bursts of high intensity. However, if properly trained, it can have great endurance. If it enjoys exercise, this Saturn tends to take it very seriously and may need to lighten up with movement that makes it feel happy. Strengthening and mobilizing the back and spine is immensely important for injury prevention.

Uranus in Leo

Uranus in Leo may experience irregular electrical sensations in the chest and spine, such as heart flutters, arrhythmia, and shooting pains or spasms in the mid back. The thyroid may have some relation. Bursts of cardiovascular exercise may help relieve pent-up electrical static. This Uranus is prone to sudden overheating and rapid depletion of the Sun's nutrients. It needs copious water and perhaps occasional high doses of magnesium and vitamin D.

Neptune in Leo

A Leo Neptune may need extra Sun and Fire-generating nutrients such as iron, protein, magnesium, vitamins D and A, and various B vitamins. Its heart and blood pressure may be slightly weak, possibly contributing to a general feeling of faintness. Because of this, Neptune in Leo may be disinclined to exercise, but promoting circulation and strength, especially of the back, will help fortify it.

Leo Nourishment Checklist	Leo Movement Checklist
Gesture: Heart(h) Food	**Gesture:** Heart Tending
✦ Colorful vegetable focus	✦ Back strengthening
✦ Daily decadence	✦ Chest opening
✦ Heart opening and protecting	✦ Joyful and mood boosting
✦ Solar nutrient focus (magnesium, vitamin A, vitamin D)	✦ Spine mobilizing
	✦ Varied cardiovascular work

SAGITTARIUS

Sagittarius Anatomy

Sagittarius is commonly compared to a wildfire because of its unrestrained, quick-changing nature. This sign's heat erratically swirls up and out in all directions. Being both mutable and Jupiter ruled makes Sagittarius enthusiastic and interested in consuming life in as many ways as possible. Its major body rulership, the legs, symbolically and physically expresses this sign's desire to explore. Sagittarius is the seeker, the wanderer, and the traveler, and its anatomy is designed to move it toward a destination. Sagittarius is where the central and peripheral nervous systems meet and where impulse turns into action.

Mode	Ruling Planets
Mutable	Jupiter

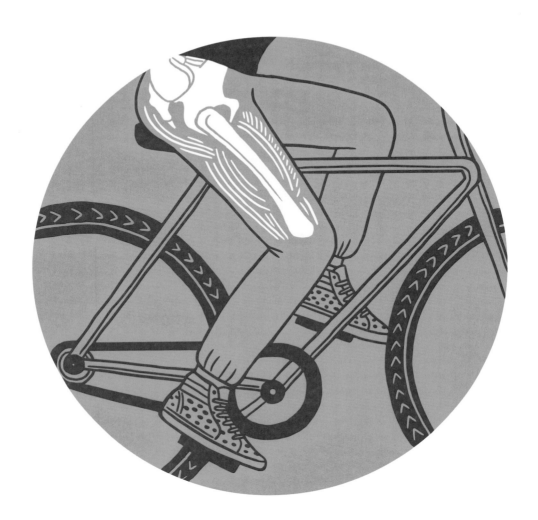

+ Muscles of the hips, thighs, and glutes

+ Pelvis, sacrum, and coccyx (with Scorpio)

+ Femur

+ Sacral nerve plexus and sciatic nerve

+ Lower spine and spinal cord (with Leo and Libra)

+ Arterial system (with Leo)

+ Liver (with Jupiter and Virgo)

+ Functions of the brain's left hemisphere including judgment and reasoning

Sagittarius Nutrition

Gesture: Exploration

Just as Leo's centripetal energy magnetizes us to its center, Sagittarius's centrifugal force inspires us to push outward and explore our limits. Sagittarius is the sign of the nomad and adventurer, and it brings its seeking nature into the kitchen. Classic Sagittarian food is an exciting fusion of cultures and flavors, sparing no expense and prepared with a haphazard touch. My Nana is a double Sagittarius, and she passed her astrological cooking genes down to me. We're multitasking, messy, and intuitive cooks. We use every appliance at once, never measure anything, maybe set a fire or two, but the meal always turns out divine.

To keep Sagittarius interested in nutrition, it's got to be exciting. Eating the same thing every day will not do for this curious sign. Luckily, healthy eating doesn't have to mean boring. Sagittarius is nourished by sights, flavors, and smells outside of the norm. Remember this when you're meal planning and grocery shopping. Make shopping a fun and expansive experience by frequenting bustling outdoor markets, global food fairs, and local farms. While you're there, pick up a vegetable or ingredient you've never used before. Keep the inspiration going and mimic these vibrant environments at home by clearly displaying colorful spices, herbs, and bulk ingredients in glass jars or containers. Sagittarius lives for experience, and it can meet this need nutritionally by eating in uplifting spaces. Sagittarius's body and soul are nourished by eating outdoors. Invest in some outdoor seating, a fire pit, or a great picnic basket.

We see Sagittarius's love of experience and stimulation in its body rulerships. Sagittarius is a major player in nervous system health. It's a very physical sign, ruling most of the muscles and nerves in the legs, but it also governs our higher cognitive ability. When healthy, Sagittarius can take lofty ideas and concepts and bring them down to earth. Proper nutrition allows Sagittarius to see clearly and take aim. But without this support, its brilliant enthusiasm and resources often go to waste because of poor planning and concentration, overcommitting, or extreme effort in the wrong direction. Sagittarius frequently expands beyond its energetic capacity. When this happens, it can experience a unique combination of mental exhaustion and global nervous system fatigue and pain. To prevent this, but still support Sagittarius's big vision, nutrition should be nerve building, brain clearing, and inflammation modulating.

Although all signs may suffer from anxiety, Sagittarius is the most likely to experience a buzzy, unsettled agitation in the mind. For this sign, the line between excitement and nervousness is microscopic. Because Sagittarius flies so high and travels so far, it needs to make sure it starts from a grounded place and with a full tank. Of all the Fire signs, Sagittarius may require the most energetically heavy diet. This usually means higher amounts and denser forms of protein and fat from eggs, well-sourced dairy, and even organ meats. Sagittarius needs a large amount of Jupiter-ruled nutrients, especially fat-soluble vitamins (A, D, E, K), essential fatty acids, and nervous system-supporting vitamin B_6. Nuts, seeds, oils, avocado, coconut, eggs, high-quality dairy, poultry, and fatty fish are Sagittarius helpers.

Supporting Sagittarius Digestion

Just like this sign's glyph, Sagittarius energy is like an arrow, always flying up and out. Sagittarius spends a lot of its physical energy thinking about the future. But to keep it digesting well in the present, it needs to come back to its lower body rulerships. Begin meals by coming out of the higher mind and into the lower body. Wiggle your hips and toes and feel where your body makes contact with the chair. Improve Sagittarius digestion even further by taking a light walk or stretching out your hips, hip flexors, IT band, and lower back after meals.

It's also important for Sagittarius to know how specific foods interact with its nervous system. Instead of relating to foods as "healthy" or "unhealthy," try relating to them as tools that are stimulating or soothing. This is highly individual, and keeping a journal noting which foods excite or soothe your nerves can be helpful. If you need some focused nervous system healing, reducing stimulating foods may be warranted for a time, but eventually, you'll be able to leverage all foods with wisdom. For example, if you know a certain food gives you an energetic boost and a sharp mind, use it early in the day and save your soothing foods for evening.

Nerve-related hip, low back, and leg pain are very common for Sagittarius. Like the other Fire signs, sometimes a personalized anti-inflammatory approach may be helpful. Never forget that Sagittarius rules both the higher mind and the lower nerves, meaning they're intricately connected. Foods (and food thoughts!) that aggravate one will aggravate the other, and foods that nourish one will nourish the other. Personalize your anti-inflammatory approach with the stimulating-versus-soothing food exploration mentioned above. If you're feeling agitated, temporarily removing your personal stimulating foods may calm both the mind and the limbs.

If pain is a large part of your Sagittarian experience, it may also be worth investigating any liver involvement. The liver, which is ruled by Jupiter, gets waste products ready to leave the body, and when its function is sluggish, we can feel heavy and burdened. Because Sagittarius rules some of our largest muscles and structures, poor liver function often expresses as pain. You can help open and smooth the liver's function by eating cruciferous vegetables and dark bitter greens, especially chervil, endive, and dandelion, which are associated with both Jupiter and Sagittarius. Digestive congestion—particularly distention, gas, or constipation—may also contribute to Sagittarian lower body pain. The structures of the lower GI, pelvis, and hips are quite close together, and congestion in one can push and prod on the others.

Sagittarius Movement
Gesture: Locomotion

Sagittarius movement reflects its freedom-seeking, exploratory nature. Sagittarius is happiest on the frontier, and it must always have the illusion of freedom, especially when crafting movement habits. As a systems-bucking Sagittarius rising, I know a thing or two about this. It's common for us Sagittarian people to jump from thing to thing. We get really interested and enthusiastic about one sport or practice, only to drop it a few months later and pick up the next shiny thing. I eventually wised up and realized I needed to give myself a consistent rotation of shiny things, meaning my routine needed to be highly variable to keep me interested and engaged. But as a trainer, I also know that moving haphazardly without intent doesn't work.

Head to clairegallagher.co/bodyastro for video examples of Sagittarius movements.

This is one of the many reasons why I developed my astro-fitness methods. I needed a mutable but intelligent system that consistently varied in intensity, movement approach, and modality.

Sagittarius isn't too interested in the details. It's more of a conceptual, big-vision sign. If Sagittarius has a basic map, it can get to the target in many different ways. In fitness, this means giving yourself an overarching program concept but allowing yourself the flexibility to fulfill it in a way that feels fun and inspiring in the moment. There are infinite ways to do this, but let's choose an easy example. One overarching training concept could be to hit cardio, strength, and flexibility work all in one week. How and when you do this is up to you and your Sagittarian whim. One week you may feel like doing classic weightlifting for your strength work, but maybe a yoga sculpt class sounds more exciting the next week. If there's an overarching concept, give yourself the freedom to play and follow your impulse.

Another pillar of Sagittarius movement is locomotion. This sign likes to cover a lot of ground. Remember that major Sagittarius themes include travel and exploration, not to mention its physical role in connecting impulse with action via the legs. Any type of outdoor movement—trail running, mountain biking, skateboarding, roller skating, skiing, obstacle races—or any destination athletic event that fulfills your wanderlust is absolutely Sagittarian. I've been known to drag all my weights outside for a backyard session (yes, even in the snowy Maine winter). Sagittarius will do almost anything for a great view and a good story. But because Sagittarius is such a forward-momentum sign, it tends to move only in the *sagittal* plane. (Interesting etymological connection!) Movements in the sagittal, or longitudinal, plane take us forward or backward. Running, cycling, walking, and squatting—classic Sagittarius movements—are all done in the sagittal plane. But to be well rounded and safe from injury, all bodies, but especially Sagittarius ones, need to supplement their sagittal motion with lateral and rotational movement (the frontal and transverse planes)—more on this in the following sections.

Beneath all of this is a commitment to lower body mastery. The legs and glutes are Sagittarius's structural domain. If I had my way, every day would be leg day—most Sagittarian athletes would agree. This rulership is certainly a double-edged sword. Sagittarius can experience both its greatest strength and greatest pain in the lower body. A well-rounded Sagittarius program accounts for this and focuses not just on lower body strength but also the balance between legs, pelvic positioning, hip mobility, and nerve care.

Sagittarius Strength and Conditioning

A classic Sagittarius strength and conditioning program will be very squat heavy. If you have a lot of Sagittarius in your chart, this type of program may feel fulfilling, but without proper technique and variation, it can cause a lot of lower body issues over time. Most Sagittarius people are quad dominant with weak glutes and hamstrings, which leaves the low back vulnerable to injury. For movement longevity, I encourage all Sagittarius-dominant people (myself included) to not only spend time mastering lower body movement mechanics but to focus double time on glute and hamstring strength. Always do a glute activation circuit before any squat work. To protect Sagittarius bodies, we want our squat to be a bit more booty and hamstring focused. Because we sit on our glutes all the time, we can feel a little disconnected from them, and they can be hard to recruit during a squat. Isolating and activating the glutes before a squat session or run can help us mentally reconnect to these vital muscles.

Be sure to branch out from the classic lifts and incorporate traveling, pivoting, and movements that change direction in your strength routines. This brings Sagittarius's movement gesture, locomotion, into the gym. Remember, you want to incorporate all three planes of motion. If you can get in two at a time, that's even better. There's a ton of room for creativity here, but a few ideas are rotating squats and lunges, traveling kettlebell swings, lateral lunges, and lateral step-ups.

Sagittarius Running

As the celestial centaur, almost any type of running will do for this sign, but the running program that leaves you feeling free and buoyant has Sagittarius stamped all over it. You know the runner's high, where you feel like you're soaring? That's the Sagittarius zone. This isn't a feeling you can force; it just tends to happen. But you can encourage it with good music, a great view, and varied terrain. Sagittarius gets bored easily. Explore new parks, trails, and neighborhoods regularly.

For a varied Sagittarius running split, be sure to give your body areas some extra challenge with stair or hill training. While hill sprints could certainly work here, unlike an Aries sprint, Sagittarius intervals are a little longer and a twinge less serious. Make sure to keep it fun. Be sure to incorporate some lateral movement and pivots into your running routine too. For some Sagittarius flair, work on side shuffles, basketball suicides, or even agility drills (like you might see on the soccer or football field). Jumping over logs and rocks on a trail run is another great way to train agility.

Sagittarius Yoga

The Sagittarius yogi craves vibrant movement like the other Fire signs but also has a deep desire to connect with the divine. Sagittarius is the zodiac's philosopher, and it's often attracted to crossovers between spirituality and movement. Yoga that builds some heat but also offers connection with a greater force or global cause often speaks to Sagittarius.

Sagittarius flows are naturally lower-body focused. Any class that offers combined hip opening, sacral alignment, and leg strengthening is a sure bet for this sign. And don't forget to make time for yoga nidra. It may not feel like a natural choice for Sagittarius, but this deep relaxation practice is extremely restorative for the nervous system.

Other Sagittarius Sports and Classes

+ Adventure and destination races

+ Archery

+ Cycling and spinning

+ Dance cardio class

+ Exotic yoga retreats

+ Freestyle dance

+ Horseback riding

+ Leg- and glute-focused classes

+ Roller derby

+ Soccer

+ Spiritual fitness fusions

+ Trail running

+ Walking

Sagittarius Conditions

Sagittarius conditions arise from both unrestrained and unfed Fire. This sign experiences immense levels of heat in the legs, nerves, and mind. This can be energizing and inspiring, but if this Fire isn't given limits or outlets, it transforms into aggravation, restlessness, and a constant whirring in the mind. Sagittarius tends to be overly optimistic about its capacity to do, and when it asks too much of itself for too long, the Fire eventually burns out. This is when Sagittarius may feel very un-Sagittarian and experience deep exhaustion, chronic pain, or feeling completely cut off from inspiration, personal freedom, and interest in the world. Sagittarius conditions may manifest as:

Accident proneness (especially the lower body)

Burnout

Discontentment

FOMO (fear of missing out)

High blood pressure

Insomnia

Low back, hip, and sacral pain and misalignments

Mental illness (usually tending toward grandiose, hyperactive, manic, or restless states)

Mobility issues

Nervous exhaustion

Pelvis or leg fracture

Poor concentration

Restless leg syndrome

Sciatica, piriformis syndrome, and similar nerve-related pain

Spinal cord injury, compression, or infection

It's natural for a Jupiter-ruled sign such as Sagittarius to expand, reach, stretch, and test its edges. I view this expansion as neutral, not good or bad but rather the standard operating mode of Sagittarius. It's not something you want to limit, but it is something you want to direct. Most suffering for this sign comes from expanding in an unskillful direction. For example, Sagittarius magnifies Fire, whether expressed as joy or rage. This sign can vigorously expand into any state of being, and because Sagittarius is a mutable sign, it may even flash between them rather rapidly. It can experience high highs and low lows in a short span of time. The most important skill for Sagittarius to learn is how to aim, direct, and take responsibility for its expansive nature.

As you navigate the world of food and fitness, compassionately remember your tendency to test the limits of things. In the early years of wellness exploration, this is easy to spot, usually looking like ferocious seeking. Expect to be drawn to flashy ideas, far-out philosophies, and intense immersion experiences. Expect to feel very passionately about one thing, only to feel limited by it later. Expect the cycle of enthusiasm, restlessness, dissatisfaction, boredom, and then reaching for something new. If you ride this cycle unconsciously for years, you'll likely wake up one day exhausted and not any closer to your destination. But if you participate in the cycle with curiosity and openness, it has a lot to offer.

As you can guess, one popular Sagittarius stereotype is that it doesn't follow through. But as a Sagittarius rising who's followed through on most things, sometimes to my detriment, I'd like to give this a creative spin. What Sagittarius might register as restlessness, boredom, or flakiness may actually be clues that your body and mind need a break or that you don't have the resources needed to continue on at this moment. It doesn't always mean you're on the wrong path and should look for something new. Usually these feelings are signals to temporarily expand in an opposing direction. As far as Sagittarius expands outward, it must expand inward. As deep as it reaches into work, it must reach into rest. As intensely as it exerts, it must receive. And as much as it consumes, it must empty out. When Sagittarius practices this, that uncomfortable itch to seek, run, and "free" itself quiets down. Plus, this tends to protect Sagittarius from burnout and exhaustion.

Pro tip: Chasing enthusiasm doesn't tend to support long-term Sagittarius health either. Believing you should always feel enthused about a workout or just life in general is a lot of pressure to put on yourself. A wise Sagittarius will check its enthusiasm just as frequently as it checks its restlessness.

Of course, sometimes a change is truly warranted. Just make sure you're clear on what's underneath the impulse before you act. Otherwise, the root problem is likely to just take on different skin. Whether it's a new workout regimen, social engagement, material object, class, relationship, or just your phone, always pause to ask, "Why am I reaching?" Compulsively reaching outside of itself is the biggest clue that Sagittarius needs to pause and regroup.

Other Planets in Sagittarius

Mercury in Sagittarius

For Mercury in Sagittarius, more than any other Sagittarius placement, mental health hinges on nutrition. This Mercury is very creative but prone to high-flying states of nervousness and agitation. Pay close attention to which foods speed up or slow down the mind. Ideally, food should feel like a grounding brain hug, full of nerve-building fats and proteins.

This Mercury has a great need for motion and can process a lot of nervous agitation through walking, running, or using the legs in any other way. It's prone to nerve pain in the hips, thighs, and low back and must slow down enough to learn proper movement mechanics or pain is likely to become a chronic issue. Because this Mercury is so restless, one of its biggest pitfalls is hopping from one workout program to the next.

Venus in Sagittarius

Venus in Sagittarius is all about experience. It loves a good party or weekend trip, and nutrition may take a backseat to its social life or whatever's most exciting in the moment. Boring food is the fastest way to lose this Venus's interest. But nourishing food never needs to be boring. To stay interested, things must be flavorful and engaging. Make gathering and cooking food an exploration and incorporate new ingredients and recipes regularly.

Venus in Sagittarius always makes me think of disco dancing. No matter what your opinion on disco, if this Venus had its way, working out would be more like a rave. (Dance cardio, anyone?) Again, this Venus bores easily, so give yourself plenty of movement variety while still upholding a larger vision. And don't underestimate the motivational power of a colorful outfit and great music. If hip, leg, or back pain is present, it's often due to a lack of strength in the surrounding structures. More stretching isn't the way to address Venus's pain. A good place to start is investigating any strength discrepancies between the quads and the glutes.

Mars in Sagittarius

Mars in Sagittarius burns through food, nutrients, and body resources rapidly. It often needs more protein, calories, and more frequent meals than other Sagittarius placements. It's also a quick responder—if you eat something that doesn't agree with you, it's likely to show up as anxiety, poor concentration, insomnia, restlessness, or pain in the hips and legs.

This Mars is rather accident and injury prone. In true Sagittarius fashion, it tends to get hurt while playing a game or goofing off. To prevent injuries, warm-ups are nonnegotiable. Because it's easily activated, it's best to schedule workouts earlier in the day so that they don't interrupt your sleep. This Mars is optimistic about its athletic ability and needs to watch its work-rest balance both within a single routine and an entire program.

Jupiter in Sagittarius

Jupiter in Sagittarius is all about freedom. Anything new can excite it, including the latest food craze, but as soon as its freedom feels squeezed, its interest plummets. If Jupiter can relate to food as something that enhances its growth and adds to its freedom, it's more likely to have a positive relationship with it. Nutrition, like all of life, is a journey and it's allowed to grow and change with you. Side note—the liver may need some extra nutritional support.

Jupiter in Sagittarius can draw up some grand plans and this often goes for fitness goals as well. If this Jupiter doesn't meet its objective, it's not for a lack of enthusiasm or vision but usually a lack of proper planning. This Jupiter knows where it wants to go, but it may need some help with the day-to-day steps. Don't be afraid to hire a knowledgeable coach who can support your big vision by working out the details.

Saturn in Sagittarius

Rather than having an expansive and exploratory relationship with food, Saturn in Sagittarius often struggles with believing it's okay for food to be pleasurable and fun. It may feel scared to venture out and try new things or cling to someone else's food "truth" and dogma instead of trusting its own. On a purely physical level, this Saturn may need assistance with fat digestion from digestive bitters or enzymes.

Saturn in Sagittarius may have experience with poor circulation, lower body fractures, hip and spinal misalignments, arthritis, or weakness in the legs. It's important to mobilize and bring as much blood flow and openness to the glutes, hips, and thighs as possible. Depression, disappointment, and feeling stuck are usually helped by moving the legs. Sometimes this Saturn is fearful of vigorous exercise and may limit itself to modalities that never challenge it or break a sweat. But it's just as likely for Saturn in Sagittarius to be overcommitted to a lofty goal that asks it to reach beyond its limits.

Uranus in Sagittarius

Like Mercury, Uranus in Sagittarius needs food and movement to act as grounding and nerve-buffering tools. Therapeutic use of oils and fatty acids may help soothe any nerve pain, spastic energy, and frenzied mental states. The lower body is prone to injury and nervous irritation, but heavy leg use is beneficial because it acts as a discharge pathway for electric agitation in the body or mind.

Neptune in Sagittarius

If Neptune in Sagittarius isn't properly nourished, the physical and mental experience may feel rather rootless and out of body. Grounding foods high in nerve-building fats and proteins are essential. Be aware that Neptune may use food to alter or escape a confining mental state. In fitness, the lungs may need intentional strengthening with regular cardiovascular exercise, and any lower body pain is likely due to glute or leg muscle weakness.

fire bodies

Sagittarius Nourishment Checklist	Sagittarius Movement Checklist
Gesture: Exploration	**Gesture:** Locomotion
✦ Denser fats and proteins	✦ Glute activation
✦ Food as adventure	✦ Leave room for spontaneity
✦ Lower body connection at meals	✦ Lower body mastery
✦ Jupiter nutrient focus (vitamins A, B_6, D, E, K)	✦ Traveling and pivoting moves
✦ Stimulating/soothing food lens	✦ Use all three planes of motion

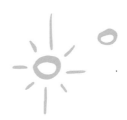

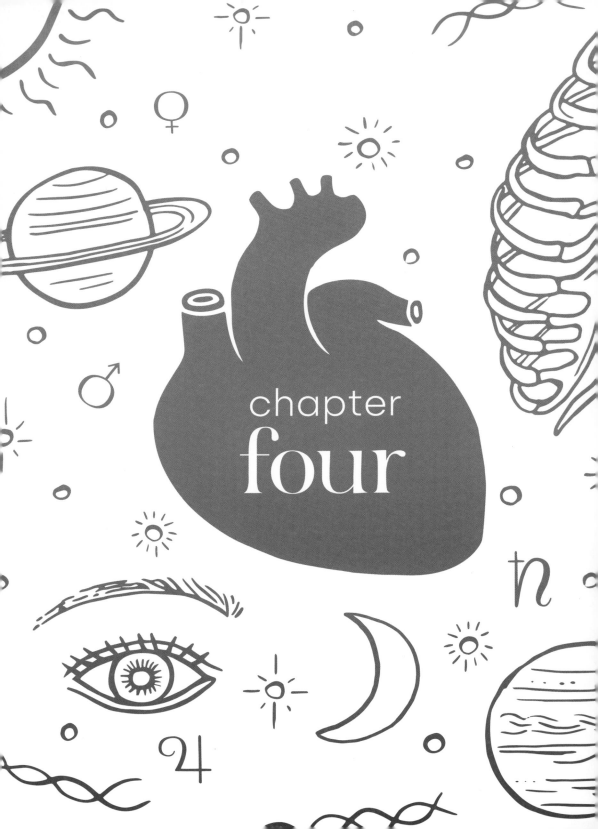

chapter
four

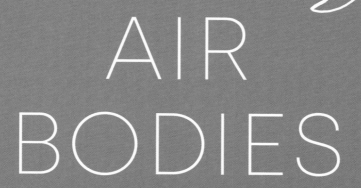

AIR
BODIES

Signs: Gemini, Libra, Aquarius
Qualities: Hot, Moist

Air reveals itself through relationship. It's invisible and unknowable outside of its interactions with the outside world. We experience Air by watching what travels through it or by receiving it. We see Air when wind rustles the leaves, carries birds and bugs, or stirs the ocean. We receive Air through sound, smell, and breath. We experience its constant motion and constant relating to the other elements as weather. Air's behavior is complex and erratic. Sometimes it's a breeze, sometimes a hurricane. It can be light and spacious or heavy and humid. It can have a single direction or feel too spontaneous to understand and predict.

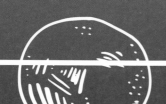

In Western astrology, Air's qualities are hot and moist. While these qualities teach us about Air's basic behavior, always leave room for its many variations. We've all felt a cold wind from the north or a dry wind from the south, and we have experienced humidity in all kinds of temperatures. Air can have many qualities. But what its traditional qualities tell us is that its original job is to quicken and combine. Heat speeds things up, and moisture melds things together. Air is a speedy connector. From here, it's easy to see why Air is associated with communication, both in the world and in the body. Hot air moves up and out, like the energy of spring, a fresh idea, a rush of blood, laughter, gossip, or a viral video.

Air is associated with any part of the body that sends or receives information. The nervous system exchanges messages with the outside world. The lungs receive oxygen and send out carbon dioxide. The vessels send out fresh blood and receive weary blood, while tons of other tubes connect organ to organ. Speaking, hearing, and processing all sensory information is a function of Air. And just as the atmosphere tries to create equilibrium by moving from high pressure to low pressure, the Air element governs the balance between body systems and gases.

Air gets into trouble when it sends and receives too much, too little, too fast, or too slow, or maybe gets the wrong message altogether. When Air moves too quickly, we may feel anxious, forgetful, or flighty. When Air is overabundant, we may feel full and bloated or spacy, like a brain floating outside of our body. When Air is slow or we don't have enough, our circulation may be poor and we can feel cold, fatigued, and deflated. People with a lot of Air in their birth chart may feel as though their symptoms come and go like the wind or that their lifestyle follows the breeze's erratic pattern. The food and movement recommendations for Air signs are meant to create steadiness while still giving Air plenty of room to fly and fluctuate.

Supporting Air Nutritionally

Remember that astrology and the body are dynamic, and you could have too much, too little, or neutral Air at any given time. Eating to support your Air may look different throughout your life. Whether it's days, months, or years apart, you may find yourself cycling through periods of eating to decrease or increase Air.

AIR NUTRITION

Decreasing Air	Increasing Air
Dairy	Alliums (chives, garlic, leeks, onions, shallots)
Frequent meals	Any foods with a naturally bright or rich green color
Iron-rich animal protein (beef, chicken, turkey, sardines)	Carbonated and sparkling water
Mineral water	Cruciferous vegetables (broccoli, cauliflower, kale)
Nonanimal blood-building foods (beets, dark leafy greens, deep-red vegetables, molasses, pumpkin seeds)	Fresh, fragrant, green herbs (basil, dill, mint, oregano, parsley, rosemary, thyme)
Nuts and seeds	Fresh fruit and vegetables juices
Oils, dressings, and sauces	Leaves, sprouts, and shoots
Root vegetables	Lightly steamed or raw food
Sea salt	Plant fats (coconut, olive)
Well-cooked, warming food	Poultry
Whole grains (brown rice, quinoa)	

Foods and Practices That May Disturb Air
Anything that gives you uncomfortable gas and bloating
Eating in front of electronics
Endocrine disrupters (such as BPA, pesticides, phthalates, phytoestrogens)
Excess caffeine
Oils used above their smoke point

GEMINI

Gemini Anatomy

Although all Air signs have a role in body communication, Gemini's is the most obvious and external. Because it's mutable and ruled by swift Mercury, it's extra speedy, extra curious, and extra flexible. The Gemini body explores the outside world and rapidly reports its findings. Gemini's anatomy isn't too interested in judging what it's carrying—it's just the messenger.

Mode	Ruling Planet
Mutable	Mercury

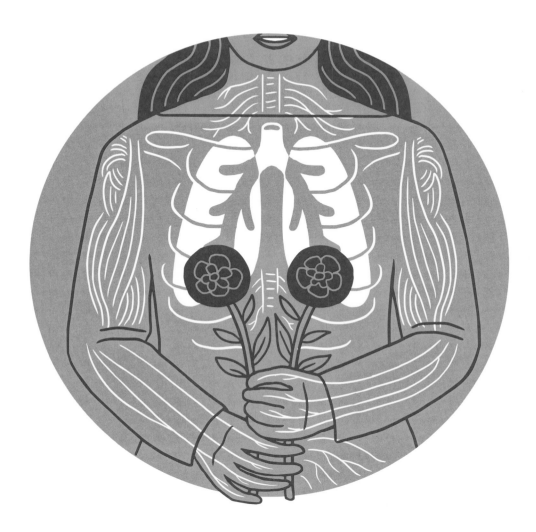

+ Peripheral nervous system

+ Clavicle, scapula, humerus

+ Upper ribs

+ Trachea, upper lobes of lungs and tubing of lungs

+ Muscles and nerves of shoulders, arms, wrists, hands and fingers

+ Capillaries

+ Tubes, tunnels, ducts, canals (bronchi, carpal tunnel, Eustachian tubes, fallopian tubes, trachea, vas deferens, ureters, urethra)

+ Speech and hearing (with Taurus)

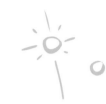

Gemini Nutrition

Gesture: Adaptable

In astrological nutrition, I'm interested in optimizing a sign's natural qualities with food. I never want to make Gemini less Gemini but rather a more streamlined and potent Gemini. Gemini is like a bird or bumblebee, quickly fluttering from place to place, gathering what's delicious and then moving on to the next thing. Gemini tends to get a lot of grief for being changeable, when its adaptability is actually its greatest strength. We want to support Gemini's flight so that it's more efficient and so that it's gathering and doing what's truly important and for its highest good. This means creating a nourishment practice with a basic pattern that is still highly adaptable and easily altered to match Gemini's current fancy.

Gemini loves variety, and when we're crafting body-supporting habits, we want Gemini to know that variety can come with it. The one constant for this sign is change, and contrary to popular belief, change and health can certainly coexist. This sign's routine is to be different day to day, moment by moment. Forcing it to be otherwise is forcing it to live outside of its essence, which never leads to true health. Adjust your surroundings to fit your essence. Don't adjust your essence to fit your surroundings. As a Gemini body, expect your food mood to change rapidly and don't judge it as a problem. Real problems arise when you're in midflight, almost out of gas, and don't have anything to catch you. Flexible nourishment is what will serve Gemini. This means a variety of foods, diverse flavors, endless combinations, glorious colors, and the freedom to consume when, where, and how you like.

But before it can truly take off, Gemini needs to create some basic nourishment habits. Once these are solid, Gemini can morph and change to its heart's content, always knowing that its nourishment habits will step in as a safety net when needed. One such habit might be stopping regularly to do a quick body scan. A common Gemini food frustration I see is the classic crash-and-burn. Gemini can get really interested in whatever's in front of it and may not realize it's hungry until ravenous and uncomfortable. Food healing for this sign almost always coincides with mental and nervous system reprogramming, where Gemini learns to pause and then read and respond to its subtle signals appropriately. When distraction, poor concentration, low productivity, nerve pain, headaches, or anxiety begin to creep up, it's time to land and refuel. These signals don't exist to confine Gemini but to prompt a refresh, so that it can go out and fly again.

Supporting Gemini Digestion

The best way to support Gemini digestion is to give the mind and nerves a break. When you're eating, just eat. Do your best to eat screen-free. This is often hard for Gemini, but probably its most supportive practice. Instead of fluttering externally, flutter internally and have fun noticing the hundreds of sensations happening in your body as you eat. Begin meals with a quick breath practice. Gemini rules inhalation. Take a deep breath in, expanding your belly, and hold for five to ten seconds; let it out with a big open-mouthed sigh. Do this three times.

Gemini can also set itself up for higher mental flight with what it puts on its plate. Ideal Gemini nourishment fortifies the nerves and brain and supercharges mental activity. This usually means a foundation of energetically lighter fats and protein and then smart carbohydrates for a turbo boost as needed. Fill your plate with foods that make you feel alert but that give you lasting fuel. Gemini wants to soar, and heavy, large meals may make it uncomfortable. Although different for everyone, plant fats, lots of green foods, and lighter animal proteins are often on Gemini's list of supportive foods. Regardless of the latest fad, find the unique food timing and dose that truly supports your performance. It doesn't have to look like anybody else's. If you struggle with the Gemini crash-and-burn effect, try pairing carbohydrates with fat and/or protein for a smoother energetic experience.

When deeper healing is needed, sometimes we must create space for the nervous system to unwind by temporarily removing overstimulating foods and beverages. For Gemini (and all signs for that matter), conscious food removal is not the end goal but a way to free up bandwidth for mental and nervous system healing. Once this foundation is laid, Gemini can usually tolerate any and all foods in moderation. Mature Gemini teaches true food freedom: there are no "good" or "bad" foods, and any food coming from the earth is valuable. You can also support Gemini's nervous system by making food planning and shopping less stressful. Gemini isn't one to make a huge menu and shop for it all at once. It's more likely to go to the market a few times per week or even daily. But for optimal nervous system functioning, Gemini needs a loose plan. Give yourself permission to only plan and shop at intervals that feel doable—every three days is a good Gemini pace.

You can also support Gemini food freedom by setting up your pantry and menu for endless adaptability. Gemini excels at adapting what I call "blank palette" foods to fit its current tastes. A blank palette food is something with a base recipe that you can change and morph endlessly, depending on what you're craving in the moment. Examples are congee, kitchari, soup, oatmeal, smoothies, granola, meatballs, stir-fries, toast variations, cauliflower any-thing—there are thousands. Prioritize having your blank palette staples on hand and then head to the store for whatever produce or twist ingredients you need to fit your current food mood. Once Gemini gets down the basic pat-tern, it'll be a master food juggler and creating homemade meals will become fast and easy—another Gemini nutrition staple. This sign often prefers prep methods and kitchen gadgets that work ultrafast or that allow it to focus on other things.

Gemini Movement

Gesture: Playful

Just like Gemini nutrition, Gemini movement celebrates and refines its adapt-able nature. Like a breeze, Gemini floats from here to there, pivoting swiftly. All mutable signs can be sloppy (yes, even Virgo) or masterful in their muta-bility. The way Gemini approaches exercise will enhance one side or the other. Although Gemini fitness may look like fun and games on the surface, a mas-terful Gemini athlete is never scattered, but instead is an expert in diversity. This is accomplished through multidirectional movement, complexity, mental engagement, and intelligent movement variety.

In exercise, it's common to move in one direction. Running, walking, squats, lunges, and push-ups all confine the body to a single track. Like its sign pair Sagittarius, Gemini reminds us that all planes of movement are valuable. When we overdevelop one direction or motion, we're left vulnerable and weak

Head to clairegallagher.co/bodyastro for video examples of Gemini movements.

when suddenly asked to move in a new way. Gemini movement is multidimen-sional and challenges the body to maintain its integrity and strength in any creative and strange position Gemini may find itself in. Imagine the dexterity of a world-class tennis player or a football running back. They consciously train their multidimensional expertise and abilities to jump, pivot, accelerate, and decelerate rapidly.

Mental engagement and movement complexity are also Gemini fitness pillars. We see this in multistep movement combinations, very high-skill and technical movements, and sports that require advanced hand-eye coordination. Don't forget that Gemini rules the arms and hands, so any sports or movements that recruit these areas and also require quick sensory processing are Gemini ruled indeed. If Gemini isn't mentally stimulated by its workout, it'll lose interest. If technical sports aren't your thing, and you're feeling stuck in your movement practice, hit up a group class or recruit a buddy. Social connection is one of Gemini's major motivators.

Remember that Gemini rules the lungs, respiratory tubing, and blood capillaries, meaning that breathing and cardiovascular training have big roles to play too. Astrological energy expresses on a spectrum. For Gemini, this could mean that heavy breathing feels natural and comfortable for some, while others struggle with poor breathing mechanics or exercise-induced asthma. For both ends of the spectrum, learning to use breath as a stabilizing force in exercise is extremely important. Whether it's bracing the abdomen for a heavy squat or controlling the breath during a yoga flow, the breath is Gemini's ticket to mastery.

Gemini Strength and Conditioning

A well-designed Gemini strength and conditioning program is fluctuating but functional. Like the other mutable signs, Gemini craves stimulation and variation in its training approach. Doing three sets of ten squats is the fastest way to lose this sign's attention. Instead of just squatting, put your feet in staggered positions, use uneven weight, add bounds or pivots, and incorporate rotation. My favorite Gemini focus is functional training. Functional movement essentially prepares us for real-life situations, such as picking up your cat, reaching and twisting for the top shelf, or carrying groceries up the stairs. Functional movement is not only fun and mentally engaging but it also trains the body for variety. Incorporate single-limb strength work, cross-body movements, and asymmetrically loaded moves—for example, single-leg deadlifts, woodchoppers, and lunges with one dumbbell overhead and one by your side. This type of training also forces Gemini to slow down, think, and be fully present with what's in front of it. In conditioning, I ask Gemini to catch some air and challenge the lungs with plyometric and explosive training. Some popular examples are squat jumps, tuck jumps, and clapping push-ups.

Gemini Running

Although I have no doubt there are Gemini marathoners in the world, this sign's energy is best expressed in track-and-field events that incorporate running, jumping, and throwing—the long jump, high jump, pole vault, hurdling, and discus, to name a few. Off the track, freerunning and parkour may pique

Gemini's interest. Even if you're a dedicated distance runner, incorporating some Gemini play into your routine will make you faster and more powerful. Don't worry, you don't have to catch too much air to reap the benefits. Incorporating side shuffles, depth jumps, backpedaling, and acceleration and deceleration drills will do the trick.

Gemini Acceleration Drill: Falling Starts

The acceleration phase is the initial portion of a sprint. The falling start is a popular drill that teaches runners how to accelerate while holding their body at the proper angle. As the name implies, you're going to "fall" into your sprint. Stand tall with your feet close together. Lean your whole body forward, keeping your ankles, hips, and shoulders in alignment. When you've gone as far as you can, fall into your sprint and rapidly accelerate for about ten meters. Give falling starts a try at the beginning of a run or as part of a sprint workout. How many falling starts you do is up to you, but begin with a set of ten with recovery time in between.

Gemini Yoga

A balanced Gemini practice will support the hands, arms, nervous system, and lungs. Pranayama (yogic breathing) and other types of breathwork practices are perfect medicine for this sign. Because it's easy for Gemini's nervous system to get overstimulated, I suggest slower breathing practices that create stability and evenness. One of my favorites is the box breath, where the inhale, exhale, and the space between them are even. For example, inhale for four counts, hold the breath in for four counts, exhale for four counts, and hold the breath out for four counts. As you get comfortable, you can lengthen the breath. Beyond the lungs, spend time attending to the strength and mobility of the wrists, hands, and arms. Arm balances are something Gemini often loves to work on, along with exploring aerial and other types of yoga that suspend you in the air.

Other Gemini Sports and Classes

- ✦ Boxing
- ✦ Break dancing
- ✦ Fencing
- ✦ Frisbee
- ✦ Group classes and movement meetups
- ✦ Gymnastics
- ✦ Handball
- ✦ Hang gliding
- ✦ Juggling
- ✦ Racquet sports (tennis, table tennis, racquetball)
- ✦ Skydiving
- ✦ Softball and baseball (especially pitching)
- ✦ Trapeze
- ✦ Volleyball
- ✦ Windsurfing

Gemini Conditions

Most Gemini conditions occur when there's a kink or blockage in its information network. Gemini's information highways include the nerves, blood vessels, and airways. A pinched nerve, cold hands, and shallow breathing are all examples of Gemini meeting trouble. However, in our modern world it's more common to see an overwhelming amount of data streaming through the Gemini channels. This can leave the Gemini body feeling distracted and on edge. Gemini conditions may present as:

Anxiety

Ear infection, tinnitus, hearing loss

Lung issues and infections of all kinds (asthma, pneumonia, bronchitis)

Nervous digestion

Peripheral neuropathy

Pins and needles, numbness, weakness, and nerve-related pain in shoulders, arms, hands, wrists, or fingers

Poor blood circulation and oxygenation

Poor breathing habits

Sensory processing disorders

Speech and language disorders

Gemini's mental game is exceptionally strong, and it tends to overthink most things, including health. At the root of many food and movement issues is a lack of clarity. This isn't because Gemini doesn't have the answers but because it tends to turn away from its own answers to seek someone else's. Gemini is a gatherer, and there's absolutely nothing wrong with this. But when Gemini turns away from its internal knowing too frequently to collect more and more information from the outside world, its own path forward can become unclear. Information overwhelm tends to either trap Gemini in a mental loop, where there's all thinking and no doing, or scatter its energy and dilute its efforts by doing too many things at once.

When Gemini energy is trapped in a loop, mind-chatter volume is turned all the way up, and it may feel consumed with options, worry, memories, fears, or just noise—like a song or a radio jingle you can't get out of your head. When Gemini is stuck in the mind, action is left behind. In fitness or nutrition, this is the difference between thinking about a workout and doing a workout or thinking about a meal and cooking that meal. Trapped Gemini furiously flutters in place, cycling its information, creating even more agitation.

Scattered Gemini energy may look very busy and action-oriented when it's actually doing everything except the one thing that needs doing. In food and movement, this might manifest as hopping from thing to thing and approach to approach. This is the fastest way to get nowhere. But it could also look like asking for everyone's opinion but your own. Remember that Gemini rules the peripheral nervous system. It's as though this sign has little tentacles constantly scanning its surroundings. Leave it to Gemini to ask for a list of books, a good article, or the latest research. And while being informed is extremely important, when you find yourself defaulting to your friends or social media for advice before asking yourself, it's a sign to reel those little tentacles back in. Commit to scanning your internal environment as often as you scan the external.

Whether Gemini feels trapped or scattered, the answer is rarely, if ever, to tell the mind to shut up. The mind's job is to inform us. It's not doing anything wrong by sharing its thoughts. Instead, stepping out of our chatter is often, quite literally, a physical step. Next time the chatter comes on, try putting both hands right below your clavicles, on your upper lungs; take a breath and ask your body, "What's the next step?" Notice I said "ask your body"—not your mind. Whatever bubbles up first, even if it's as simple as "Take a sip of water," do it. Then, ask again. And again. Expect the mind to balk and tell you how worthless this is. But even small actions, done consistently, will create big clarity and cultivate trust in your lived experience. For Gemini, clear information is always preferable to more information.

Other Planets in Gemini
Mercury in Gemini

Mercury in Gemini is curious, mentally busy, and may forget to eat and drink at regular intervals. Dips in blood sugar or hunger and thirst may masquerade as nervousness or anxiety. Avoid getting to this point by setting a gentle alarm as a reminder to pause regularly for a quick body scan.

Exercise can be a welcome thought organizer and cleanser for this planet. Give yourself a good combination of routines that require absolute presence, as well as those that allow you to mentally zone out. Don't neglect upper body strength, and pay extra attention to shoulder and wrist mobility to prevent the upper body nerve pain commonly experienced by Mercury in Gemini.

Venus in Gemini

For Venus in Gemini, a social butterfly, food is a vehicle for chitchat. This Venus is the type to throw a great brunch and wind up hungry because the conversation was much more exciting than eating enough. The food mood changes frequently, and Venus in Gemini tends to shop as the desire and need strike. This may get a Gemini Venus into trouble because it's prone to fluttering blood sugar. Nutritional issues may show up as skin conditions on the arms and hands or as respiratory reactions.

Just like food, exercise is often another opportunity to mingle. Venus in Gemini loves to play, and fitness may take the form of games, matches, and walks with friends. Sometimes there's more play than work, but Venus doesn't usually mind. The upper body is vulnerable to pain, but most of this can be prevented or remedied with appropriate strengthening and postural therapy.

Mars in Gemini

Mars in Gemini is one of the speedier metabolizers of the zodiac. The nervous system consumes a lot of energy and may benefit from more frequent, stabilizing meals. Mars in Gemini may be aggravated by air pollutants and prone to respiratory conditions that are hot and urgent in nature. Be curious about foods that may contribute to lung strain, such as dairy, sweets, and greasy or poorly sourced meat.

Much of the time, Mars in Gemini is a natural athlete. It often enjoys that out-of-breath feeling and may be drawn to highly cardiovascular sports that allow it to travel and explore, such as running or cycling. Like most planets in Gemini, this Mars is prone to pain in the arms and shoulders, but instead of weakness, it's often due to overuse, injury, or accident.

Jupiter in Gemini

Jupiter in Gemini carries the essence of a hot-air balloon and may need nutritional support to stay tethered to the earth. It needs a combination of light and grounding foods such as root vegetables. High-quality fats and minerals are also necessary to soothe the nerves and give this sometimes excessively buoyant Jupiter a few boundaries.

Jupiter in Gemini thrives on large amounts of fresh, clean air, and like other planets in Gemini, it may be more attracted to aerobic exercise. This is important to keep up because the lungs and circulatory system are Gemini health priorities. But to keep this Jupiter from flying too high, it must incorporate some weight-bearing work. Plyometric and weighted explosive movement could be a fun compromise.

Saturn in Gemini

Saturn in Gemini often needs help circulating air and blood through the body and relaxing the nerves. A balanced, nutrient-dense diet that focuses on circulation-supporting foods such as beets, cayenne, cinnamon, garlic, onions, and turmeric may be helpful. Pay close attention to your posture and breathing, as well as the air quality, during meals. Nutritional issues and food reactions may manifest as arthritis-like pains in the arm, wrists, or hands.

Saturn in Gemini is associated with a stuck or restricted feeling in the lungs and chest. Within movement, this may show up as asthma, exercise intolerance, or simply poor breathing mechanics. A supportive exercise program may include mindful breathing techniques and methods for gradually increasing lung capacity. Postures that reverse blood flow, such as inversions, may be helpful as well.

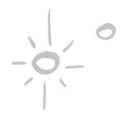

Uranus in Gemini

Like Mercury in Gemini, Uranus in Gemini is tightly wound and prone to nervousness, stress, and neurological conditions. It may find stopping to take care of its physical needs to be a little annoying, but regularly timed food and movement keep this Uranus out of the crash-and-burn zone. Rhythmic breathing and upper body mobility are important movement focuses.

Neptune in Gemini

Neptune can bring weakness to Gemini's body, whether it's the lungs, arms, nerves, or cognition. Neptune in Gemini may feel like it doesn't have enough air, and it may help to "oxygenate" the body with bright, fresh, green food. Mixed cardio and controlled breathing intervals may be very helpful with lung capacity—for example, running in place for a minute, followed by a few rounds of box breathing (see page 104). This Neptune is very sensitive to air pollutants, so do your best to exercise in a clean and clear environment.

Gemini Nourishment Checklist	Gemini Movement Checklist
Gesture: Adaptable	**Gesture:** Playful
✦ Nervous system support	✦ Multiplane, diverse movement
✦ Heed subtle body signals	✦ Hand-eye coordination
✦ Embrace your food mood	✦ Functional fitness
✦ Create an adaptable pantry	✦ Lung strengthening
	✦ Social motivation

LIBRA

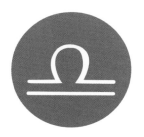

Libra Anatomy

Libra's primary physical function is to maintain the body's equilibrium. We tend to think of balance as a static state, but it's an extremely dynamic function that requires constant coordination and tweaking. Maintaining homeostasis is a multiorgan process, with a lot of filtration, distillation, secretion, and excretion. Libra governs many interconnected cycles and complex feedback loops. Although it may not look like much on the outside, Libra's "balance" is a continuous rising and falling of blood, water, and hormones.

Mode	Ruling Planet
Cardinal	Venus

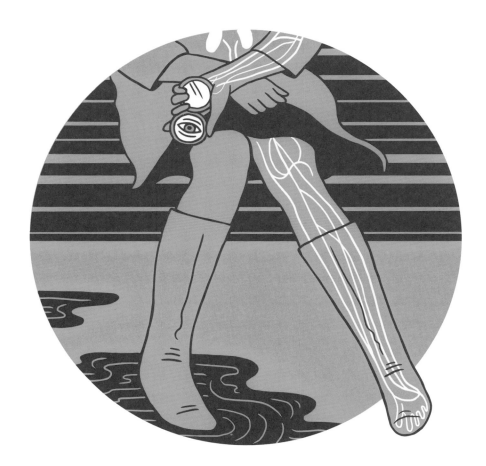

+ Homeostatic mechanism (the coordination of many organs and includes blood acid-base balance)

+ Kidneys

+ Adrenal glands (with Aries and Mars)

+ Urinary bladder, ureters, and urethra (with Scorpio)

+ Lower back muscles, lumbar spine, and lumbar nerves

+ Ovaries and testes (with Scorpio)

+ Fallopian tubes (with Gemini)

+ Veins (with Aquarius)

+ Complexion

Libra Nutrition

Gesture: Balance

No matter where you live in the world, Libra time occurs at an equinox, either autumn or spring. This is the moment of the year when light and dark are equal, and where Libra's association with balance originates. Libra governs the transitions between all polarities—dark to light being just one. Even its glyph reminds us of a sunrise or sunset. Light and dark can't exist without the other, and mature Libra values both sides of any polarity equally. Balance is a really hot word in the health space, and I find it's often used in a way that creates shame—as though we're always just out of reach. But Libra models that balance is an ever-churning cycle, not a strenuous straddling of two sides. Supportive Libra nutrition allows you to define and have confidence in your own experience of balance, independent of external approval, and leaves space for that experience to change over time.

Defining nutritional balance for yourself begins by noticing where you've internalized external health judgments and giving yourself permission to question them. You may be surprised, but disordered Libra eating expresses a lot like Virgo. One of Libra's symbols is the judge, and instead of developing a neutral food voice, it's often eager to cling to systems that categorize or moralize food, such as counting points, macros, calories, or adhering to lists of "free" foods and "cheat" foods. This may feel fine for a short time, but ultimately separates you from true Libra power: knowing that you can trust your own food desires, tastes, and preferences without moving into mental or physical discomfort.

Let's make up a polarity. On one end is the food you want, and on the other, the food you think you "should" have. When Libra rejects what it wants for what it deems more "acceptable," it'll eventually experience a boomerang effect. This could express as reactive eating, compensatory exercise (where you "work it off"), or another type of self-punishment. Libra clients often tell me they have no self-control or willpower when it comes to food. If they know some astro, they might even crack a joke about being Venus-ruled (the planet of pleasure). But this loss-of-control feeling around food usually stems from long-term deprivation from Venusian pleasures because of an assumption that it will make them more lovable, acceptable, or righteous. And if they *do* allow themselves what they want, their inner food judge showers them with guilt, which simply drives the Libra boomerang effect deeper. Cultivating neutral food talk is a foundational step in healing Libra's food relationship.

Defining nutritional balance for yourself also means respecting your body's daily rhythms and transitions, such as sleep/wake, hunger/fullness, work/rest, and so on. But to honor these transitions, you've got to know when they're happening. When you've internalized external judgments of health for an extended period, it can be very hard to identify your own physical transitions. It can even suppress biological hunger signals! *This is not your fault.* From a nutritional therapy perspective, if you feel disconnected from your natural feeding rhythm, creating a temporary rhythm may help reconnect you. Experiment with eating consistent meals at the same time every day, even if you don't feel physically hungry, until that internal sensitivity is turned back on. This is essentially managing blood sugar, which is one of the best ways to not only keep Libra's transitions smooth, but to keep it from developing hormone imbalances and other conditions associated with this sign.

Speaking of blood sugar, because Libra is governed by Venus, it's highly attuned to both carbs and sweetness (Venus rules sugar, carbs, dairy, and fruit). This doesn't mean carbs are "good" or "bad" for Libra. Don't fear the carb! It just means Libra responds to carbs, the sweet flavor, and the manipulation of them very strongly. But if you're experiencing a Libra health condition, you may discover that pairing low-glycemic carbohydrate foods with a denser protein or fat gives you a smoother physical experience. Libra is the sign of equality, therefore consuming carbs, protein, and fat at every meal tends to be a sure bet. If you want to take this Libran plate design a step further, try getting all five flavors on your plate—bitter, salty, umami (savory), sour, and sweet. By the way—most grains and root vegetables are sweet in flavor, although your palate may not register this at first. Chew root vegetables, grains, beans, and other carbohydrates slowly and get to know their sweet taste.

Digestive Harmony

Libra digests best in a harmonious environment. Sure, it's unrealistic to expect complete control over your eating environment all the time, but do what you can to create steadiness in your body before picking up your fork. Harmony is an internal state, and just like training a muscle, your ability to cultivate it gets stronger with practice. Begin meals by placing your hands on your low back and taking a few even breaths with an equal inhale and exhale. Take a few moments to admire the colors on your plate, the smells, the way the light hits it—no matter how small, find some beauty.

Libra is more likely to make supportive food choices when its surroundings not only feel harmonious but look harmonious. My Libra mother never goes to bed with dishes in the sink—not because she's a clean freak but because she likes the feeling of sipping her morning coffee in a clean kitchen. Fill your surroundings with sweetness and you may be surprised at how it enhances the feeling of satisfaction with your food. Libra is nourished by good lighting and food that looks as delightful as it tastes. Eat meals in natural light, low light, or candlelight as often as possible. Have fun plating your food and invest in appliances, dishes, utensils, and glasses that make your heart sing.

Because Libra's such an important player in hormone balance, it's also important to be mindful of endocrine disruptors. These chemicals are found almost everywhere in our modern world, but especially in cosmetics, personal care products, pharmaceuticals, pesticides, processed food, and food packaging. One of the easiest ways to avoid endocrine disrupters in the kitchen is to get rid of plastic food containers and use body- and eco-friendly glass or ceramic containers. It's important for all signs to educate themselves and make informed choices about chemical exposure, but Libra is especially vulnerable to their effects. Do your research, read labels, and buy organic if accessible for you.

Libra Movement

Gesture: Symmetry

When Libra is awakened, it values a life that feels good. Every task, habit, conversation, meal, and even workout becomes a canvas for harmonious life design. With the right tools, Libra can become a truly poised, wise, and well-rounded mover. The underbelly of Libra is often motivated by appearances. It's easy for Libra to relate to movement purely as a means for physical alteration and skewed social elevation. If you're a Libra who values appearance, there's no need to shame this part of yourself—it's simply an aspect of your Venusian DNA. But be really careful of falling into the Libra trap of conflating "looking good" with feeling good. This

Head to clairegallagher.co/bodyastro for video examples of Libra movements.

mindset may lead Libra to shun movement altogether or engage in exhausting cycles of yo-yo exercising and dieting. Working out may always be work, but if it doesn't ultimately feel good and enhance life, it's not working for

Libra. For movement to be a Libran harmonizing tool, you need to leverage symmetry and scaling and learn to find the sweet spot.

Libra is represented by a scale, and its job is to maintain homeostasis. In a movement scenario, this means doing what it takes to create symmetry in your structure. Symmetrical structure creates more ease in the body—it feels good. Remember that finding balance is a dynamic process, requiring tons of micro-adjustments. Likewise, creating symmetry doesn't happen by doing symmetrical, bilateral movement. It happens in asymmetrical and uneven movement. Libra movement, such as ballet and surfing, looks graceful and smooth but requires a ton of balance. To develop this skill and the illusion of symmetry, Libra training methods often have to isolate and divide the body into upper and lower or left and right halves.

Libra's quest for homeostasis also teaches that we can have the best of both worlds: a training program that creates physical benefits and brings more joy to our lives. This is the sweet spot—a magical place where there's enough stress in a session or program to create growth but also enough rest for that growth to flower. Effective training challenges us but leaves us alert, inspired, and more available for the rest of our lives. Regularly take stock of your workout routine to be sure it's still contributing to your entire life balance and that it's not disrupting it. Your exercise sweet spot will never be the same as someone else's and that's where the Libran concept of scaling comes in. Workouts should have an intent. They're not haphazard but artfully designed to elicit a specific effect in the body. Our bodies are vastly different, and how we create this desired effect is relative to our fitness level and movement history. Scaling a workout allows each body to experience the intent of a routine by adjusting variables such as weight, equipment, work times, rest times, and movement complexity. Scaling a workout doesn't make it less effective but rather more effective, because it tailors the exercise dose to your body.

For example, let's pretend the intent of a session is strength endurance. Person A has been training for five years and has great squat form. I give them three sets of twenty barbell squats at a moderately heavy load. Person B has been training for six months and is just getting comfortable under a barbell. If I were to prescribe the same number and type of squats at the same weight, I'd miss the entire intent of the training session. They'd be working at their personal maximum, they wouldn't even finish the first set, and they'd get very frustrated along the way. The rest of their training week would probably get messed up too, because they'd be too sore and tired from this one session.

You can take this same idea and apply it to any movement. You wouldn't put a brand-new dancer in pointe shoes or ask a new yogi to fly up into an arm balance. There are intelligent and supportive progressions. When you don't scale, you lose the art and magic of a session. When you continue to do this over time, you overextend the body and sabotage yourself by contributing to Libran hormone imbalances. Even if you have a trainer or go to group classes, you are *always* in charge of your ability to scale. You never have to do a workout as written. It can be as simple as doing fewer reps, dropping one set, or adding thirty extra seconds of rest. Working *within* your capacity will actually support faster and more sustainable growth.

Libra Strength and Conditioning

The bulk of Libra strength work is unilateral, meaning isolating one limb or side at a time, such as in single-leg deadlifts, single-leg squats, and single-arm presses. We can create even more balance challenge by incorporating contralateral (opposite arm, opposite leg) and ipsilateral (same arm, same leg) movement. If I were to ask you to hold a kettlebell over your head with your left arm and step up on a box with your right leg, that would be contralateral. If I were to ask you to hold a kettlebell over your head with your left arm and step up with your left leg, that would be ipsilateral. Both are valuable in Libra strength training and offer the body a unique challenge. We can put a Libra spin on bilateral movements too—for example, doing squats on uneven surfaces or loading the left and right sides differently.

Also, be mindful of training muscle agonist and antagonist pairs equally. These are muscle pairs located on opposite sides of a limb, such as the biceps and triceps or the quadriceps and hamstrings. One acts as a prime mover, while the other is passive. We tend to work one harder than the other (usually the one we can see in the mirror), which can create imbalance, pain, and poor function over time. But no matter what you do in a session, the Libra intention is to leave some gas in the tank for the rest of your life. Your training should support your energy, not drain it.

Libra Running

Libra values leisure. This sign reminds us how to make space for fun in our movement practice. Whatever makes running fun, do that—whether it's a buddy, new music, a social media challenge, or training for an actual fun-run event. For you serious Libra runners, be sure to make space for leisure runs that keep you connected to your love of the sport. Also, pay attention to the strength balance between your quads and hamstrings, as well as the balance between types of terrain—for example, working on downhill running as much as uphill running.

Libra Yoga

No surprises here—a Libra flow will focus primarily on balancing postures, from Half Moon to Dancer, all the way up to advanced handstands. The low back is also an important Libra yoga focus. Sessions that focus entirely on the low back or end with restorative low-back postures are very Libra supporting. This sign often gets locked up in the quadratus lumborum, a muscle in your low back roughly spanning from the bottom of your ribs to the top of your pelvis. Side opening postures can be very helpful for this too.

Broaden the concept of balance to include the yin/yang or dark/light balance of your entire practice. Do you only practice yin forms of yoga (more cooling, calming, and restorative)? Only yang forms (more heating and vigorous)? Why do you think this is, and how can you bring them into an appropriate equilibrium?

Other Libra Sports and Classes

- ✦ Ballet
- ✦ Barre
- ✦ Bosu and balance-ball training
- ✦ Competitive bodybuilding
- ✦ Paddleboarding

- ✦ Partner sports
- ✦ Pilates
- ✦ Slacklining
- ✦ Surfing
- ✦ Tennis

Libra Conditions

Libra conditions develop when the body's continuous rising and falling loses its regularity. Too much, too little, too fast, too slow are all common Libra problems. Libra issues tend to be more complex than they appear because of the multihormone dance this sign orchestrates. When one part is off, it's likely another is too. These conditions rarely happen out of nowhere—they take time. Libra can endure quite a bit of asymmetry before an issue is perceptible. Although not always the case, Libra complaints are often traced back to living an asymmetrical lifestyle or tolerating disharmony for too long. Libra conditions may present as:

Blood sugar swings

Cortisol imbalances

Difficult fluid and blood pressure regulation

Fertility challenges

Hormonal acne or other skin changes

Hormone imbalance

Inability to regulate body temperature

Insulin resistance, poor carbohydrate metabolism, diabetes

Interstitial cystitis

Kidney issues of all kinds including poor function, stones, infections, and disease

Low back pain, weakness, spasm

Ovarian issues (cysts, polycystic ovary syndrome, anovulation)

Poor venous circulation, spider veins, varicose veins

Sexually transmitted infections

Urinary tract infections and any difficult or frequent urination

Weight cycling from chronic dieting

Comparison is one of the most common roadblocks to Libra's health. Whether it shows up as judgment, criticism, indecision, or self-consciousness, chronic comparison is a sure way to keep Libra feeling off-kilter and far from the harmonious state it represents. Libra is a relational sign, and it learns a lot from its reflection in others, but it can get stuck in a painful game of external validation and mirroring. There are infinite ways this could manifest in nutrition and fitness, such as confusing cultural ideas of beauty with value, relating to movement as a status symbol, judging your diet as better or less than your friend's, thinking everybody's watching you at the gym, neglecting your inner wisdom to follow your partner's workout routine, or enduring the migraine from a post-work cocktail because you don't want your coworkers to judge you.

Libra is a natural pleaser. It teaches us about equality, kindness, and tact. But if Libra calibrates its internal scale to someone else's, it may abandon its own needs to keep the peace or to keep up appearances. This is how the sign that's assumed to be the epitome of balance often feels and looks like the most imbalanced sign of the zodiac. Tons of physical healing can occur for Libra when it steps off the inaccurate scale of external approval and becomes its own compassionate judge.

I like to think of healthy Libra energy as a beautiful sine wave. It has evenly distributed crests and troughs, or peaks and valleys. Ideally Libra's body and lifestyle easily and naturally fluctuate. The transitions are rounded, smooth, and comfortable. It has work. It has rest. It has pleasure. It has discipline. It must be alone. It must be together. For Libra, all sides are true and valuable. But when Libra clutches to perfectionism, pleasing, or fear of not living up to a certain expectation, its bodily experience becomes a jagged roller coaster. There's so much energy being exerted to uphold this image, idea, or relationship that it is utterly exhausting. Libra may get stuck on an intense peak, in a lethargic valley, or violently waver between the two. It'll experience inverted cycles of all kinds, such as extreme work schedules, disrupted circadian rhythms, irregular cortisol curves, and debilitating swings in mood and energy. Remember that balance is a dynamic, oscillating process. Getting rid of Libra's oscillating nature wouldn't get it closer to balance. We all move through wise periods of light and dark dominance, just like the seasonal year. It takes a lot of effort to fight this. Instead, Libra healing often occurs in riding the wave. As Libra develops understanding and compassion for its fluctuations, they'll become smoother, gentler, and more dependable.

Other Planets in Libra
Mercury in Libra

In both fitness and nutrition, Mercury in Libra's constant comparing may keep it completely immobile or wavering between approaches. It feeds on intellect and can see all sides of something, including the pros and cons of any food approach or workout program. It may get stuck deliberating or perhaps obsessively weighing and measuring food and tracking how many calories it's burned throughout the day. This Mercury benefits from descending out of the mind and developing a deep relationship with its internal scale or its lived bodily experience and the physical facts.

Mercury in Libra may experience urinary irritation ranging from frequent infection to incontinence. Nerve pain in the low back is also common and may be helped by improving pelvic floor integrity and learning to activate the glutes and lower abdominal muscles.

Venus in Libra

Venus in Libra will do almost anything to keep things smooth, peaceful, and pleasant on the surface. It may chase its or someone else's idea of perfection, only to later find itself on the extreme end of a hormonal seesaw. Regularly check that you're not ignoring your physical needs to uphold an image, reputation, or perhaps the needs of someone else. Hormone imbalances are common, and Venus in Libra's nutrition ideally protects and repairs these cyclical ebbs and flows. This Venus may have a sweet tooth that ramps up during relational stress. Sweetness is therapeutic for this placement, but excess sugar may aggravate any underlying conditions.

Venus in Libra isn't typically attracted to aggressive, sweaty, loud workouts. It prefers graceful, artistic movement modalities such as dance or yoga. If it does happen to be a gym rat, it'll often make the hardest things look dance-like and easy. This Venus occasionally gets caught up in exercising to look a certain way or as a means for climbing the social ladder and may need help mending and deepening its relationship with movement.

Mars in Libra

Mars can feel a little awkward in harmonious Libra. This placement is the most likely to vacillate rapidly between the peaks and valleys of the Libra wave. It's not quite sure how to manage its energy and may overthink and procrastinate or overshoot and exhaust itself. Mars in Libra needs nutrition to be simple and stabilizing. Don't give it too many options. Nourish the adrenals and keep consistent mealtimes to help Mars stay steady. Give the kidneys plenty of water because they're prone to inflammation and taking the brunt of this Mars's stress. Food reactions may show up as uncomfortable energy crashes and surges or bladder irritation.

Because of its aggressively vacillating nature, scaling workouts is extremely important for Mars in Libra. You want to balance and sustain this Mars's energy, not exhaust it with poor workout design. Try to work out early in the day when cortisol is at its natural peak. This Mars is prone to back injury, so take plenty of time to warm up and get a slight sweat going before you begin more vigorous movement.

Jupiter in Libra

Jupiter in Libra typically loves food and often has a soft spot for Venus-ruled sugar, chocolate, baked goods, fruit, and dairy. Finding pleasure in food is an important part of this Jupiter's self-care, but so is keeping its blood sugar in check. Having dinner for breakfast is one of my favorite Jupiter in Libra tricks. It may be helpful for this planet to have a large savory meal early in the day to set a stabilizing nutritional tone for the hours ahead.

Jupiter in Libra can be easygoing about fitness. Movement that has a social component, such as team sports or a community league, might be more attractive than going to the gym. Circulation can be a bit lax, so Jupiter is wise to take plenty of walks and reverse blood flow frequently with easy inversions such as legs-up-the-wall. Cultivating low-back strength is also very important, so be sure to incorporate deadlifts, good mornings, rows, and pull-ups whenever you can.

Saturn in Libra

Roadblocks to Saturn in Libra's well-being tend to come in the form of decisions or relationships. This Saturn is prone to food- and workout-decision fatigue. Having too many options is the quickest way to exhaust it, eventually leading Saturn to grab whatever's easiest or skip food or movement altogether. Plan ahead so you don't have to make food decisions after a busy day, and know what workout routine you're going to do the night before. Simplify and ask for help if you need it. This Saturn can carry some hefty self-doubt, and getting a little sage advice for peace of mind may be helpful. Saturn in Libra often feels a strong responsibility to uphold its relationships. If this goes to an extreme, Saturn may find itself enduring poor health habits and patterns to keep everything intact.

Saturn in Libra is prone to a chronically stiff low back, often exacerbated by weak glutes. Strength work, mobility, stretching, and bodywork to open and fortify the Libra areas are often necessary. If other risk factors are present, Saturn in Libra may experience kidney stones, poor kidney function, and kidney inflammation.

Uranus in Libra

A bit like Mars in Libra, Uranus in Libra may find itself vacillating between overexertion and exhaustion. Uranus often inverts the smooth cycles of Libra, disrupting menses, appetite, sleep, and energy level. Blood sugar regulation is often the best place to start nutritionally. Uranus is prone to spasmodic low-back pain but may find more relief in strengthening the abdominals than stretching.

Neptune in Libra

Very much like Venus in Libra, the sweet flavor is therapeutic for Neptune in Libra, but it may find excess sugar in any form to be highly aggravating or fatiguing. The kidneys may be somewhat vulnerable, especially later in life. Maintain their function long term by keeping blood pressure and blood sugar in a healthy range. Aggressive movement might not be attractive to Neptune, but it may be motivated by a beautiful environment or music.

Libra Nourishment Checklist	Libra Movement Checklist
Gesture: Balance	**Gesture:** Symmetry
+ Balance blood sugar	+ Balance training
+ Consistent mealtimes	+ Contributes to overall life balance
+ Cultivate neutral food talk	+ Fun and leisure
+ Define balance for yourself	+ Low-back support
+ Harmonious surroundings	+ Scale and modify
+ Pair carbs with protein and/or fat	+ Unilateral, contralateral, and ipsilateral movement
+ Watch for endocrine disruptors	

AQUARIUS

Aquarius Anatomy

Beyond its muscles, bones, and tendons, the parts of the body governed by Aquarius are less like bits and pieces and more like fields of potential. They're those magic pulses, flashes of aliveness and awareness, that make us human. I believe, as modern science and the wisdom of traditional medicines complement and validate each other, more and more will be added to the Aquarius anatomy list. For example, let's go ahead and put the mysterious workings of the fascial network and the unseen—but very real—acupuncture meridians and chakra system on the list. If it holds a charge, pushes you beyond your anatomical boxes, is a little bit weird, and can't quite be pinned down by your randomized clinical trial, it's probably Aquarian.

Mode	Ruling Planets
Fixed	Saturn (traditional)
	Uranus (modern)

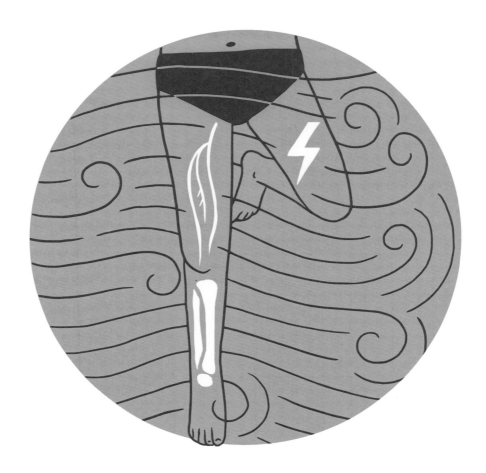

+ Muscles, bones, and tendons of the lower legs

+ Ankles

+ Venous circulation (with Venus and Libra)

+ Blood (with Pisces)

+ Oxygenation of blood and body

+ All electrical charges, ions, nodes, and currents in the body

+ Energy body (with Pisces)

+ Rods and cones of the eyes

Aquarius Nutrition
Gesture: Autonomy

You know what a heartbeat looks like on an electrocardiogram? That's a perfect example of Aquarius energy. It's choppy and jagged, but a repetitive rhythm. Each Aquarian has a unique electrical rhythm, or life flow, distinctly different from the next. Aquarius is regularly irregular. It's living contrast. This is not something to fix with nutrition but something to enhance. When you eat to enhance your unique rhythm or flow, you keep yourself humming in that Aquarian realm of electric potential where you're happiest. I like to call this realm genius.

Now, before you other signs get offended, let me be clear—we all have access to genius. But for Aquarius, connection to genius is its lifeline. The charged air before a thunderstorm, the thrilling thought that gives you goose bumps, ideas that flood your mind in the shower—Aquarius lives for this stuff. You can call it whatever you like: creativity, inspiration, flow, higher self, Source, God/dess, Science, or Universe. But without this channel, the Aquarian body withers away. Protecting your genius by keeping this channel clear is your number one nutritional priority.

Salt to Ground and Reboot

Unless you have high blood pressure, salt is your Saturnian friend. It grounds you and serves as a conductor for your electric rhythm. Become a salt connoisseur. Collect different types, colors, and flake sizes and try smoked and specialty salts. When used externally, salt reboots Aquarius by clearing external static and getting it back in touch with Source energy. Create a salt body scrub or soak in Epsom salts regularly. Pro tip: This also goes for Saturn's other sign, Capricorn.

Protecting your genius is a pretty abstract concept (typical Aquarius), so let's give it some bones. Aquarius loves to live in the mind, and it often excels there. But sometimes it can come across as a bit spacey, aloof, detached—here but not *here*. It's somewhere else, seeking that realm of genius. It gets these characteristics from its modern planetary ruler Uranus—the planet of breakthrough and progress. But if Aquarius really wants to reside in the coveted world of genius—in the realm of brilliant ideas, aha moments, and breakthroughs that actually stick and make a difference—it must pay homage to its other ruler, Saturn. What brings genius to earth? Saturn. What takes genius and makes it into a book, painting, song, medical discovery, social revolution, or new business? Saturn. What keeps Aquarius free? As odd as it sounds, Saturn—the planet of boundaries and groundedness. Are you Aquarians squirming yet? But when we put Uranus and Saturn together, we get personal authority. Personal authority is the foundation of Aquarian health and is what preserves a clear channel to genius.

Anything that creates static in this channel isn't supporting Aquarius. Static feels like many of the imbalance symptoms on page 113. But a bigger clue may be self-doubt and thoughts such as: "I have so many ideas but I never do anything with them." "I never finish what I start." "I can't trust myself." "I'm so inconsistent." So, which foods create channel static? It might not be food at all! Assigning nutritional specifics for Aquarius is not only difficult, as no Aquarian will eat the same, but it's the quickest way to create a dysfunctional food relationship. Telling Aquarius what, when, or how much to eat overrides personal authority, fuels self-doubt, and creates more static.

Personal authority includes setting nutritional boundaries, a.k.a. developing food autonomy. This means being your own expert when it comes to feeding your body. It also might mean telling a partner, family member, or even a health care provider that their comments on your body and food choices are unwelcome. It might mean telling your friend that you love them, but don't want to hear about their new diet. Food autonomy means challenging dietary rules and norms and developing your own definition of health. It also means setting boundaries around your own food thoughts. Remember that Aquarius can get stuck in the mind and will often respond to the body like a computer. Hunger may be refuted with thoughts like: "But it's not time to eat yet." Or, "I can't be hungry, I just ate." This is the mind overriding the body. Obsessive thinking and worrying about nutrition also creates static and separates you from genius. All of these things take up a ton of mental energy that could've been used on something more fulfilling or vital.

Being food autonomous may sound radical or even frightening. You may be scared you'll go into food rebellion and never come back. Take it from an Aquarius Moon who has been there—you won't. And if you do rebel for a time, remember that rebellion is a normal, healthy Aquarian response to your boundaries being violated. It's a sign to investigate where you, someone else, or "wellness" culture has overridden your personal authority. And no—food autonomy is *not* anti-health. When you approach food from a place of autonomy, you have the option to use your personal experience of static as a guide. Ultimately, Aquarius is motivated by whatever will support its genius and preserve its mental clarity and creativity. More often than not, and only after food autonomy is fully embraced, Aquarius will find that consuming nutrient-dense foods most of the time will do just that.

Channel-Clearing Meals

Treat meals as opportunities to clear static and reconnect with your inner genius. Begin meals by connecting with the aliveness of your food. Breathe in its energy, oxygen, and clarity; hold the inhale for a moment and then let it out with a big openmouthed sigh. Repeat as many times as you like. Aquarians are highly sensitive to electronic and magnetic fields (EMFs), so put your phone, laptop, and other electronics in a different room while eating. And don't pressure yourself to be social unless you want to. You never know what may flash across your brain during a meal alone.

Again, the specifics of what creates channel clarity or static will be different for each Aquarian, but it's time for my Aquarius Moon to offer a few personal observations. Channel clarity may be preserved by drinking tons of water (adding lemon and sea salt is recommended for most Aquarians), stabilizing blood sugar, keeping regular mealtimes, and eating protein (Saturn's macronutrient) and green food. Bulk prepare something each week that you can use as a quick shot of oxygen—or jet fuel back to genius. This might be green in color, light in energy, and bright in flavor. For some Aquarians, channel static may be created by food additives, dyes, and chemicals; synthetic sweeteners; excess alcohol; excess caffeine; poor food combining; erratic mealtimes; eating in front of screens; and unaddressed nutritional deficiencies (for Aquarius, it's almost always vitamin D, iron, and vitamin B_{12}). Eating food you're sensitive or intolerant to can be a big source of static too. But keep in mind that for Aquarius, the real culprit is often not the food itself but whatever's muddling it. Be curious about additives, packaging and processing residue (BPA, MSG, yellow no. 5), fruit wax, and anything vague such as "flavor." And don't forget unhelpful food thoughts and judgments! Subtle energy can disrupt Aquarius's clarity too. Don't just rinse your produce; spray or soak it in a solution of water, vinegar, and lemon juice. This isn't just about dirt or pesticides. A lot of hands touched that food and you don't have space for other people's static.

Aquarius Movement
Gesture: Pressure/Release

If all the Air signs were weather patterns, Aquarius would have the highest atmospheric pressure. This pressure comes from its fixed nature and its ruler Saturn, the planet of heaviness and restraint. But then there's the Uranian aspect of Aquarius too, giving it the need to be boundless, explosive, and free. Being Aquarian can sometimes feel very dissonant, but in truth, these qualities are interdependent, not mutually exclusive. When Saturn and Uranus combine, they create a breakthrough. Aquarius is like a spring under tension, absorbing energy to create release. The higher the tension, the more powerful the release.

We see this Aquarian imprint in sports that require an athlete to create pressure and then catapult themselves very high into the air, whether it's a slam dunk in basketball or the gymnastic vault. Because Aquarius is ruled by extreme planetary opposites, Aquarian sports often bring or expose the body to extremes. These movement modalities also tend to challenge ankle strength and proprioception, as seen in ice skating.

In Aquarius fitness, I want to train this sign's ability to break through. Without breakthrough energy in our world, we'd have no electricity, internet, modern medicine, or great works of art. Aquarius progresses humanity, but if it doesn't know how to endure tension, it's not going to progress very far. To break through to the Uranian realm of genius, you must train in Saturn's pressurized realm of discipline. In fitness, I help Aquarius master its breakthrough energy by creating environments of physical and mental tension and then asking it to free itself.

Aquarius Strength and Conditioning

In strength and conditioning, there's a ton of ways to build pressure in the body, but one of the most effective techniques is increasing time under tension, or how long a muscle is under strain during a set. In Aquarius fitness, you want to increase this time as much as you can to create that Saturn pressure, squeeze, and muscular fatigue. You can do this with long isometric holds or by slowing down dynamic exercises with a tempo. Aim for sixty to ninety seconds under tension per set. For example, ten regular-paced barbell back

Head to clairegallagher.co/bodyastro for video examples of Aquarius movements.

squats might take you twenty seconds. But if I asked you to slow down each portion of the lift—taking three seconds down, a two-second pause at the bottom, and two seconds back up—ten reps would take seventy seconds at the very least. If your weights are heavy enough, the last rep or two should be extremely hard. Tension has been built and your muscles will be burning.

But this is just the Saturn part of the equation. Once the pressure is built, you need to break through. Again, there are countless ways to do this, but an easy example is doing a plyometric (jumping) exercise immediately after your long tension-building set. This could involve doing a set of bodyweight jump squats after your seventy seconds of weighted back squats. You could also follow any isometric hold with a sprint, or pair any slow, pressure-building exercise with speed work. Other examples are resisted sprints, explosive lifts such as the snatch or clean and jerk, ballistic kettlebell movements, and weighted plyometrics. Think testing your vertical jump after doing a bunch of deadlifts, box jumps while holding a dumbbell, jumping rope with a weighted vest, or throwing a sandbag as far as you can.

Aquarius Running

To create the pressure-release effect in Aquarius running, you can use resistance in various forms. Resisted sprints are my personal favorite. You can do these by putting a resistance band around your waist and having a buddy hold it while you sprint in place as fast as you can, using a parachute, or simply doing hill sprints and allowing the terrain to be your resistance. But instead of stopping immediately after your sprint is over, drop the resistance and keep going. This is the release portion, which teaches Aquarius how to meet a limit and then break through to the other side.

Also be sure to do regular ankle mobility, calf stretching, and breaking up of any adhesions around the shinbone. Twisting an ankle is a very common Aquarius injury, as is rupturing the Achilles tendon. Your Aquarius Moon author once rolled both ankles in one race.

Aquarius Yoga

Kundalini may be the most Aquarian yogic tradition. Through challenging breathwork, chanting, and rather rapid and repetitive postures done for extended periods of time, this practice certainly builds pressure in the body. The intent is to awaken coiled or stored energy (*kundalini shakti*) at the base of the spine and bring it up to the crown of the head. This is thought to bring a breakthrough or awakening of sorts and increased self-awareness, and allow vital energy to flow freely. But it's not just the physical practice that's

Aquarian. Even the words used to describe kundalini practices, such as *technology*, are very Aquarian indeed.

Because Aquarius tends to struggle with poor circulation, yoga routines should also include plenty of inversions to assist the blood in coming back toward the heart. Even if you like to practice later in the day, start your morning with a short walk or mini movement session to get the blood pumping. Poor circulation blocks Aquarius from its personal genius, and it often feels more alert and connected after exercise.

Other Aquarius Sports and Classes

+ Basketball

+ Gymnastic floor routines

+ Gymnastic vault

+ High jump, long jump

+ Ice skating

+ Jump fitness classes

+ Oxygen-deprivation training

+ Rollerblading

+ Sports that use technology

+ Training in extreme cold or at high altitudes

+ Trampoline or rebounder

Aquarius Conditions

If this sign is anything, it's contrast. Ruled by planetary opposites Saturn and Uranus, many Aquarius conditions occur when its electric potential, energy, blood, water, or air gets stuck and then bursts through erratically and unexpectedly. Saturn contains. Uranus frees. Anything that cramps, swings, jumps, or flows backward is Uranian. Anything that's depressed, deficient, pressurized, or retained is Saturnian. These conditions often feed each other. A simple example—Saturn's fatigue and dehydration eventually explodes as a Uranian cramp. If you're Aquarian, you have the unique (but doable!) task of learning to live within your polarized anatomy, or being in your body can feel very unsmooth. Aquarius's conditions may present as:

Anemia

Cardiovascular conditions, especially electrical

Dehydration and electrolyte imbalance

Depression, bipolar disorder

Edema and swelling, water retention

Extremely variable energy, mood, mental state, or interest

Injury to, pain, or weakness in lower legs or ankles

Jumpiness, easily startled

Low blood pressure, dizziness, fainting

Multiple sclerosis

Muscle tics, spasms, and cramps in skeletal, smooth, or cardiac muscle

Nervous system overwhelm

Poor circulation (blood clots, cold hands and feet, spider and varicose veins)

Poor eyesight

Sensitivity to electronics, artificial light, sound, smell, chemicals, weather change

Sinus headaches

Social anxiety

Earlier I talked about Aquarius having a unique electrical current, or life flow, that needs to be embraced and nurtured. Aquarius energy doesn't tend to plod through the body slowly and smoothly. It's more like a jagged series of all-out sprints, punctuated by periods of withdrawal. Many Aquarius food and fitness issues arise from mishandling or suppressing this authentic flow. Authentic flow is a massive concept that touches everything from relationships to style and career choices. But in a health context, authentic flow refers to the unique patterns of your physical energy and mental attention. Maybe this pattern is backward, upside down, or counter to that wellness expert's "perfect morning routine" or the nine-to-five workday, but it works brilliantly for you. Leaning into this personal rhythm and developing habits that fit within it is when Aquarian health flourishes. If your nourishment practices go against your authentic flow, it's only a matter of time before you rebel against them or begin to feel unwell. Yes, inauthenticity is so painful for this sign that it can contribute to illness.

Aquarius typically learns to suppress its authentic flow from an early age, often when it starts school and realizes its flow is a bit different. When Aquarius suppresses its authentic flow, it experiences a loss of personal authority and freedom. Remember, personal authority isn't just a nice idea for Aquarius but a primal need. When it's stripped away, the body's alarm bells begin to ring and a rebellious, self-preserving cascade begins. Sure, some Aquarians may rebel externally, but never forget that this is a Saturn-ruled sign. Self-rebellion is just as likely. Aquarius may suppress its own flow because it believes doing so is the only way to fit in, be successful, stay healthy, keep the job, receive love, and so on. No matter what form the rebellion takes, it's a symptom of an Aquarius whose personal authority has been overridden.

This wrestle between personal authority and social norms is the complex backdrop of Aquarius health. In exercise and nutrition, this may manifest as inconsistent and choppy self-care habits, but it has nothing to do with lack of willpower. Self-sabotage and rebellion come up so frequently for this sign because, at first, developing health habits may register as an unsafe loss in personal freedom. But truthfully, if you instill healthful habits that support *your* authentic flow, they can bring you fully into your personal power and freedom.

On the other hand, maybe Aquarius rebels and preserves an illusion of personal freedom by being a fitness or dietary extremist. Being different and special is a form of rebellion too (and a nod to Aquarius's sign pair, Leo). I've done both, but as an Aquarius Moon with a Virgo Sun, my default was health specialness. In my early twenties, I practiced an extreme diet for a long time. Looking back, it's clear I wasn't choosing this "lifestyle" because it supported me and made me feel good. I was so stripped of personal authority in another area of life that dietary extremism was my way of trying to reclaim it. Once I got the help I needed and could exercise my authority in the appropriate realm, my health habits regulated.

Awakened Aquarian energy is less of a rebel and more of a purist. It's a purist in its need to be itself and live in its own flow. This self-devotion is its most important health habit. When it's solid, everything else falls into place and the yell of rebellion becomes more of a tickle on the back of your neck. It's simply a messenger, reminding you to check in with your flow.

Other Planets in Aquarius

Mercury in Aquarius

Sometimes having Mercury in Aquarius can feel like an electrical storm in the mind. It's bright and intelligent, but the inconsistency can often feel uncomfortable. Nutritional issues may show up as or contribute to stark changes in mental state. To keep this Mercury steady, it may need regularly timed nutrition. It's probably going to recoil at this idea, so start small and set reminders. This Mercury may feel best keeping an alternative working, exercising, and eating schedule. It's okay if your schedule is "irregular" and different from everybody else's, just make it *your* regular—commit to it.

Exercise can be a useful mental processing and stabilizing tool. This Mercury tends to like quick movement of the lower legs, and may enjoy jogging, skating, or playing basketball. It's important that this is balanced with plenty of single-leg strengthening and ankle proprioception work. Lower leg cramps are common. Drinking lots of water is a given and electrolyte supplementation is often necessary.

Venus in Aquarius

Venus in Aquarius often needs help oxygenating the body, and it tends to do well with an abundance of crisp, fresh, green-colored foods. Regulating the blood sugar with high protein and fiber in the morning can also help regulate any wavering interest and attention. This Venus enjoys feeling a little different and may have unique tastes in food, or if the rest of the chart is Earth heavy, it might be quite picky. It's often a very conscious consumer. How workers are treated, how food is made or grown, and its impact on the environment are important to this planet.

This Venus's circulation can be a little poor. Water retention, cold hands and feet, spider veins, varicose veins, or fatigue from lack of blood flow are possible. Although you may not feel like it, give working out in the morning a go, or at least take a brisk walk to kick-start circulation and prevent this "Air fatigue" later in the day. Prop up your feet and reverse blood flow frequently. Your ankles may be vulnerable to injury, so be sure to prioritize balance work.

Mars in Aquarius

Mars in Aquarius often feels supported by consuming blood-purifying foods, or foods that assist the liver—beets, berries, cruciferous vegetables, garlic, ginger, turmeric, and anything with a rich, green color. This Mars can be a bit defiant and may buck against keeping regular self-care routines, or it may find it difficult to accept health advice from others. No problem. Instead of thinking of nourishing habits as things that chain or contain you, try reframing them as behaviors that ultimately bring more freedom into your life.

As with most Aquarius placements, a lot of this Mars's drive and energy is in the mind, and exercise can be a helpful tool for getting it back in the physical body. This Mars may enjoy working out solo, and it tends to be more interested in quick, fast-moving routines that engage the brain rather than a jog around the block. Explosive exercise can be liberating and inspiring.

Jupiter in Aquarius

Jupiter in Aquarius is prone to bloating, gas, and other forms of pressurized air such as sinus headaches. This Jupiter is often up for trying any new, slightly weird, and alternative approach to address its concerns. It loves gathering knowledge, but often the real answer is closer to home. Personal freedom and authority are extremely important to this planet. Commit to filtering all new health information and advice through your own inner knowing before acting. Rely on the wisdom of your energetic and physical body to guide you.

This Jupiter's spirit and mental state are very responsive to exercise. Heavy breathing is especially therapeutic and can lift Jupiter out of a funk. But if all Jupiter does is cardio, it can float away like a hot-air balloon. It needs to balance itself with plenty of resistance training. Fun combos of weighted exercise and cardiovascular bursts are a good compromise.

Saturn in Aquarius

Saturn in Aquarius is prone to weak, cold blood and may need more iron, vitamin D, warming food, animal protein, and salt than other Aquarius placements. It can be quite the purist in mind and body and may have very particular dietary needs or strict thoughts and judgments around food. There may be some fear in fully stepping into its own power and authority. This can sometimes take the shape of following dietary restrictions and rules to a fault. Break your own rules once in a while.

Saturn in Aquarius often experiences stiffness, weakness, or arthritis in the lower legs or ankles at some point in its life. This is usually a consequence of long-term poor circulation, cold, or nutritional deficiencies. All facets of Aquarian fitness are needed to keep this Saturn strong but not inflexible and stubborn. Focus on ankle mobility and strength, calf stretching, and pairing pressurizing techniques with light, explosive movements.

Uranus in Aquarius

Like Mercury in Aquarius, Uranus in Aquarius's eating, working, sleeping, and exercising patterns may be viewed as highly irregular by outsiders. Although the body generally thrives on regularity, if Uranus is a prominent player in your chart, part of maintaining health also means accepting this unique pattern and allowing it to be expressed and even enhanced. Uranus is often involved in ankle and calf injury, or rupture of the Achilles tendon. Regularly stretch, mobilize, and lubricate the tendons in your lower legs and bottoms of your feet.

Neptune in Aquarius

Neptune may make the blood of Aquarius weak both in substance and circulation. Keep plenty of blood-building, mineral-rich foods on the menu. Take frequent walks and use inversion and movement breaks to keep blood and oxygen moving throughout the entire body. Keep your ankles and lower legs strong with balance work and single-leg resistance training.

Aquarius Nourishment Checklist	Aquarius Movement Checklist
Gesture: Autonomy	**Gesture:** Pressure/Release
✦ Be your own expert	✦ Ankle strength and proprioception
✦ Explore electronics-free meals	✦ Creates tension
✦ Feed your genius	✦ Opens energy channels
✦ Internal and external salt	✦ Plyometrics and explosiveness
✦ Question food thoughts and rules	✦ Supports circulation
✦ Thoroughly wash produce	

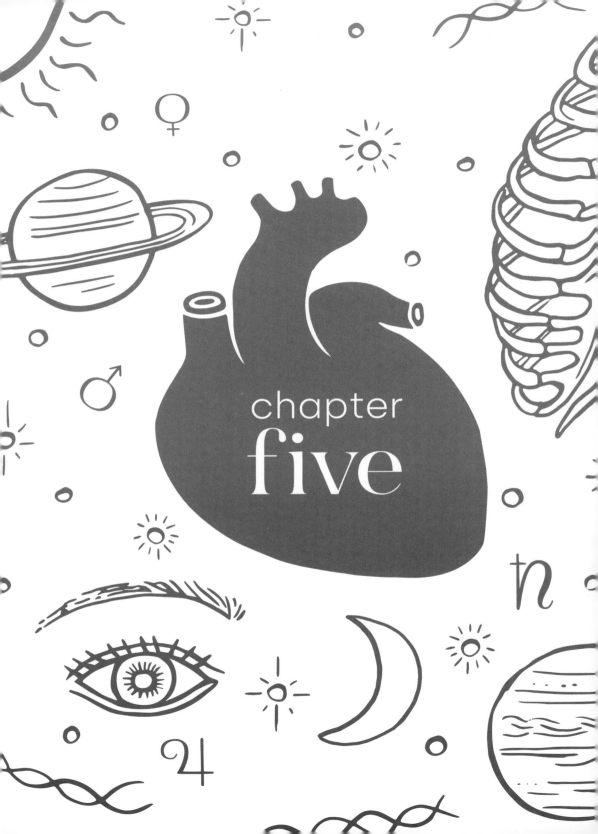

chapter
five

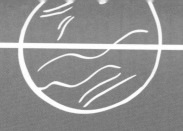
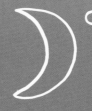

EARTH
BODIES

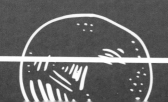

Signs: Taurus, Virgo, Capricorn

Qualities: Cold, Dry

To understand the Earth element, we simply need to look beneath our feet. In astrological theory, Earth is cold and dry, but there are many types of Earth in nature. Some Earth is certainly cold and dry, but some is warm and fertile, or sandy, or rocky, or covered with wildflowers. Plants and trees are also a form of Earth. The words *cold* and *dry* indicate Earth's energetic purpose, which is to create a solid place for us to build our lives upon. Earth supports, shelters, and feeds us.

Cold and dry also hint at what the three Earth signs rule in the body. These signs oversee all the hard structures that keep us upright, protect us, and give our flesh some shape. Other Earth body parts allow us to receive nourishment from our food, which clearly comes from the Earth. Earth gives the body strength, structure, stamina, and nutrition.

If you have an Earth-dominant body, it's often vital to replicate the Earth's stability and regularity in your self-care and lifestyle. Earth bodies thrive when they feel safe and secure, and when they can see themselves in the natural patterns of the world around them. Caring for an Earth body is typically very practical and rhythmic. These people are highly attuned to the physical plane and often need to reconnect through complete embodiment via the senses—tasting, smelling, seeing, hearing, and feeling, as well as making and crafting. After all, one of Earth's superpowers is manifestation, and everything we know is a result of it.

Wealth, abundance, and fertility are also essential Earth concepts. The Earth is rich. Its minerals, oil, and metals create kingdoms and status. Beyond security and safety, Earth bodies thrive by cultivating a deep sense of self-worth and value. Of course, this wealth is ultimately sourced from within, but it's also highly healing and nourishing for Earth bodies to interact with abundance, money, physical objects, and resources without shame.

Supporting Earth Nutritionally

Remember that astrology and the body are dynamic, and you could have too much, too little, or neutral Earth at any given time. Eating to support your Earth may look different throughout your life. Whether it's days, months, or years apart, you may find yourself cycling through periods of eating to decrease or increase Earth.

EARTH NUTRITION

Decreasing Earth	Increasing Earth
Fresh herbs (parsley, rosemary, sage, tarragon, thyme)	Broths, soups, and stews
Fresh lemon and lime juice	Collagen
Leaner forms of protein (fish, poultry)	Dairy
Lightly cooked and steamed food	Denser forms of protein (red meat, fattier cuts)
Low-carbohydrate vegetables (asparagus, broccoli, cauliflower, dark leafy greens, zucchini)	Natural sugars (honey, dates, maple syrup)
Warming spices (allspice, cardamom, cinnamon, cloves, cumin, mace, nutmeg, star anise, turmeric)	Nonhydrogenated plant fats and oils (avocado, coconut, flaxseed, olive)
	Roots, squashes, and tubers
	Salt
	Simple, well-cooked food
	Soaked or sprouted grains, legumes, nuts, and seeds

Foods and Practices That May Disturb Earth

Nonnutritive sweeteners and sugar alcohols (agave, aspartame, erythritol, high-fructose corn syrup, sorbitol, stevia, sucralose, xylitol)

Commercial corn

Excessively fatty animal protein

Gluten-containing grains

Large amounts of hot herbs and spices (excess garlic, excess ginger, horseradish, hot curry blends, hot paprika, hot peppers and chilies)

Raw cruciferous vegetables (broccoli, cauliflower, kale)

TAURUS

Taurus Anatomy

The Taurus body areas can be divided into two major categories: the things that allow us to interact with pleasure, beauty, and the physical world and rhythmic structures that create steadiness and regularity in the body. Taurus Earth cradles the brain, keeps the head upright, and regulates our metabolism and temperature via the thyroid. But Taurus is also ruled by the planet Venus, the primary indicator in astrology of pleasure, sensuality, love, and sweetness. Venus enriches Taurus with these qualities and correlates it with the senses, which allow us to experience the pleasures of life.

Mode	Ruling Planet
Fixed	Venus

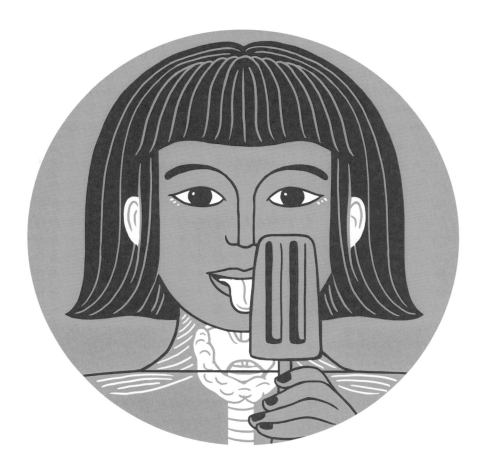

+ Occiput

+ Cerebellum

+ Ears

+ Jaw

+ Tongue

+ Lower teeth

+ Cervical vertebrae, neck, and upper trapezius

+ Throat and vocal cords

+ Thyroid gland

+ The senses

Taurus Nutrition

Gesture: Pleasure

Taurus nutrition supports regular body rhythms and steady energy circulation, but it also leaves ample room for pleasure and satisfaction in eating. When Taurus is nutritionally sated and its energy, emotions, and digestion are circulating freely, it's extremely constructive and unstoppable. To keep Taurus moving, focus on balancing blood sugar, increasing fiber consumption, and nourishing the metabolism.

Taurus is ruled by Venus, the planet of sugar, starch, and carbohydrates. All Venus-ruled signs have a sugar story and, beyond loving a sweet treat, Taurus's story typically involves blood sugar regulation. Because of the fixed, accumulating nature of this sign, high blood sugar is more common than low, although both are possible. Either way, Taurus may find it feels most stable consuming higher amounts of protein and fat in comparison to carbs. I encourage my Taurus clients to try beginning their day with a savory meal that's high in protein and fat. A quick egg-and-veggie scramble with avocado, a sweet potato-spinach-sausage hash, or even dinner leftovers are just a few ideas. This keeps energy humming and sets the nutritional tone of the day. Eating savory food early in the day often gets the taste buds (ruled by Taurus) ready to reach for nutrient-dense foods later on. Setting the tone gives Taurus a nice push in the right direction, and once momentum builds, it tends to stay on course.

Venus and Carbs: A Love Story

Planets rule macronutrients. Saturn and Mars rule protein, Jupiter rules fat, and Venus rules carbohydrates. Because they're Venus ruled, both Libra and Taurus are sensitive to carbs. I don't mean they have a carbohydrate intolerance (although that's occasionally possible), or that carbohydrates are "good" or "bad" for them, but that carbohydrates have a significant effect on their body and mood, whether more pleasant or unpleasant. These signs often need to be more mindful of what kinds of carbs they consume and how they make them feel. It's also important for Taurus and Libra to think critically when it comes to food talk that villainizes carbs, instead allowing themselves to make up their own minds based on their own physical experiences. A few of my favorite carbs for Venus signs include sweet potato, winter squash, and legume-based pastas. And when making a sweet treat (Venus signs need to live a little!), opt for nutritive sweeteners such as honey, maple syrup, molasses, or fruit.

~~~~~~

Again, thanks to sweet Venus, Taurus typically adores food. Pleasure is a pillar of Taurus health, but so is moderation. For long-term health, finding where pleasure and nutrition intersect is a Taurus priority. Balanced Taurus meals are simple and earthy but rich in flavor, experience, and love. It's like an abundant farmers market full of textures, smells, colors, and sounds. Taurus may love a decadent meal, but in daily eating, something as simple as upgrading dried herbs for fresh can satisfy this Venus-governed sign. Use as many local, farm-fresh ingredients as possible to add an element of daily decadence, and don't fear fat. Barring any food allergies, using real butter, real cheese, real sugar (yes, I said it!), and whole eggs satiates Taurus and often keeps it from indulging elsewhere.

No matter what Taurus is eating, pleasure and nutrition can be increased tenfold by how it's eating. Although it tends to eat fast, slowing down the food experience with table settings, candles, music, and conversation is immensely healing for this sign. Even something as small as drinking your morning coffee out of the cutest mug in the cabinet is good Taurus nutrition. Get your senses involved and make cooking a joyful, full-body experience. Taurus doesn't only feel nourished by tasting but also by seeing, feeling, smelling, and hearing the scenes of the kitchen. Because Taurus rules the lower teeth and jaw, chewing is also a part of this sign's food healing. This includes the classic advice to chew slowly and completely, but because it's common for Taurus to have difficulty chewing, this also means addressing pain patterns in the jaw or face and any underlying emotions that may accompany them.

Taurus digestion can sometimes feel slow and retentive. Experiment with food timing and energetics that keep you well fed and sustained but feeling open. You may find that smaller, more frequent eating or longer spaces between meals create this feeling for you. Just be sure that you're getting enough total calories. Another helpful Taurus opener and energy circulator would be fiber. Increased fiber helps improve and regulate gut motility and motion, which is often where Taurus hits a roadblock. The best Taurus fiber sources are vegetables and beans, but if you need help increasing your fiber consumption, try creatively incorporating psyllium husk, chia seed, or flaxseed. All three of these are easily added to smoothies, oatmeal, granola, puddings, and baked goods. Sipping on hot lemon water, herbal tea, broth, or other warm beverages throughout the day is another Taurus trick.

Although not true for all, hypothyroidism may affect a handful of Taurus-dominant people at some point in their lives. The thyroid is like the body's thermostat, and when it's sluggish, things slow down. Hypothyroidism, even subclinical, is often at the root of other Taurus symptoms such as slow metabolism, fatigue, and constipation. If you need more targeted thyroid support, increase iodine, zinc, and selenium-containing food such as seaweed, fish, eggs, and Brazil nuts. Reducing foods high in goitrogens may also be necessary for a time as they can block normal thyroid function. But if you choose to experiment with this, I encourage you to work with a practitioner, as many goitrogen-containing foods are also very nutritious. Some common goitrogen-containing foods are cassava, cruciferous vegetables, soy, strawberries, and sweet potato.

Taurus Movement

Gesture: Slow and Steady

Taurus movement keeps the body's rhythms consistent by supporting metabolism. Taurus excels at slow, steady work that's done over long distances or periods of time. Taurus athleticism is less about getting a cardiovascular rush and

Head to clairegallagher.co/bodyastro for video examples of Taurus movements.

more about slowly accumulating warmth. When wanting to rev the metabolism, most people go straight to high-intensity cardio, but Taurus teaches us a better way. An often overlooked part of metabolism support is NEAT, or nonexercise activity thermogenesis. Increasing your NEAT is as simple as taking the stairs, gardening, doing chores, using a standing desk, or parking farther away from the store entrance. Simply moving more during the day is very nourishing for Taurus health.

The other major way to support metabolism long term is to build lean muscle mass. Lean muscle mass is metabolically active, which means it uses more energy, even at rest. But we don't build lean muscle mass doing cardio. When working with Taurus-dominant people, I typically advise them to swap their current ratio of cardio and strength work. For example, instead of doing cardio three times per week and resistance exercise once, I want them to focus on strength three times per week and do cardio once. All zodiac signs need cardiovascular exercise, but a Taurus body tends to feel more supported with increased strength work.

Sometimes it can be difficult for Taurus to get started with an exercise routine. This makes sense considering the sign's fixed energetics, but it's totally workable and can be transformed into an asset. Taurus may take some time to warm up, but it tends to have a tipping point. Once this sign gets over the initial habit-forming hump, momentum takes over. It's equally hard to stop a Taurus as it is to start a Taurus. When first starting out, it's important to remember that regularity is part of Taurus's success formula. Too much variety and change could overwhelm Taurus at first. Consistency is way more valuable for this sign than extremes and complexity. It's wise to start with a weekly routine that's repeatable and that gradually progresses over time. In the day-to-day, if you feel sluggish and unmotivated to work out, just commit to doing a warm-up. Once Taurus gets warm, it typically wants to continue.

Taurus Strength and Conditioning

Taurus weightlifting is simple and straightforward. Choose a classic strength program that focuses on the major lifts (squat, deadlift, press) at high loads, with plenty of rest between sets. Although lifting weights in any capacity can condition the body and make beginners stronger, true strength work is done with low reps (five or less per set) and high weight. Whether lifting heavy or moderate loads, put in heavy effort. Safely flirt with failure at the end of each set while still maintaining good form. Choose weights or repetition amounts where the last two to three reps are very hard. If you don't need about two minutes of rest after your strength sets, that's a clue that the weight or reps need to be adjusted.

If you don't want to lift super heavy, no problem. You can create a Taurus effect using moderate weights and training tools such as movement tempos, pauses, pulses, and holds. These tools put the body under tension for longer periods of time and are very effective at building strength and muscle. Tempos are movement time prescriptions, just like a metronome in music—for example, taking three seconds to come in and out of each squat. Slow, controlled movement is extremely challenging. Resistance bands are another fun way to insert Taurus energy into any sweat session. Whether used alone or in addition to weights, bands add that classic Taurus stick-in-the-mud feeling to any movement and require greater stabilization and concentration. If you want to add some variety to your strength work, play with some other Taurus equipment such as chains, stones, hammers, tires, yokes, sandbags, and sleds. Anything that requires you to plod, crawl, drag, pull, or push is very Taurean.

Taurus Running

Taurus is nourished by the natural world, so take your runs outside—or better yet, to the forest—as frequently as possible. As a fixed Earth sign, Taurus will most likely be drawn to long, slow distance running. This is wonderful for Taurus, but it's important that you change things up occasionally or this sign can get stuck in a rut. I talked about resisted sprints in the Aquarius section (another fixed sign), but resisted running is my favorite way to challenge Taurus without asking it to move too fast. This exercise will be less of a run and more of a slog or march. For example, take a jog in a weighted vest or rucksack, or, if you have access to one, pull or push a weighted sled in your yard or a local field. Long nature walks and hikes are also great complements to a Taurus running program.

Taurus Yoga

Slow practices that focus on long posture holds are more Taurus's style. This could include long restorative postures, but also challenge yourself with extended standing and balancing poses. Remember, for Taurus, slow doesn't necessarily mean easy. Slow is often where Taurus builds the most fortitude. Regularly incorporate appropriate stretching, self-massage, and care for the Taurus body areas, including the upper shoulders, neck, jaw, and occiput. A practice environment that gets the senses involved with music, plants, sacred objects, and responsibly sourced incense often keeps Taurus inspired and committed.

Other Taurus Sports and Classes

+ Ax throwing

+ Cross-country running

+ Cross-country skiing

+ Football

+ Hiking

+ Mud runs

+ Powerlifting

+ Power walking

+ Rucking

+ Strongman training and competitions

+ Yardwork

Taurus Conditions

From body to spirit, the most common Taurus complaint is feeling blocked. Taurus is a fixed Earth sign, which means it moves through the world in a steady, solid, and unchanging way. These are valuable Taurus qualities unless the Earth becomes too rigid or muddy and brings life to an uncomfortable halt. A Taurus body will most likely communicate imbalance through stagnant physical and mental states or an inability to create steadiness in the body. Imbalanced Taurus loves to accumulate and hold on to things, even if those things or behaviors become toxic and self-sabotaging over time. Burying pain, holding a grudge, or any other form of psychological gripping and grasping keeps the body's energy from circulating freely and may contribute to the symptoms and conditions listed below.

Blood sugar dysregulation	Sinus congestion and infection
Constipation	Sore throat, tonsillitis, voice loss
Earache and ear infection	Temporomandibular joint (TMJ) syndrome
Emotional repression	
Fatigue accompanied by feelings of body heaviness	Thyroid conditions
	Toothache
Neck pain	

Taurus clients often report that their number one health challenge is "indulgence." Although on the surface this may appear as reaching for more food or alcohol, it often requires a deeper exploration. Indulging restrictive thought or behavior patterns, such as what we might see in orthorexia or exercise obsession, is just as common. Indulgence isn't defined by what's being consumed but how. It's a behavior loop where consumption has become compulsive. Regardless of what Taurus is compulsively consuming—food, drink, television, exercise, or thoughts—the behavior imbalance is the same.

When Taurus is in an indulgent pattern, it's usually a signal of disembodiment. As a Venus-ruled sign, Taurus feels satisfied and nourished when inhabiting the physical body. Satisfaction flowers out of fully experiencing something, and full experience requires presence and embodiment. When Taurus is missing this sensory depth and connection, compulsive consumption keeps it in a dissatisfied search for more. When Taurus expands its idea of what it means to be satisfied and allows itself to be fed by all the sensory experiences around it and within it, compulsive consumption gradually heals.

Stagnation is another common Taurus experience. This is an uncomfortable slowing or blocking of flow in the body, mind, spirit, or life. It can come from many things, but for Taurus, stagnation is often a product of long-term compulsive consumption, refusal to transform past emotional hurts, or stubborn attachment to one way of exercising or eating, even if it's causing harm. Taurus's flow is naturally slow and relaxed, but when it's completely blocked, everything begins to back up and accumulate, creating mental and physical pain. It may take years, but when things build to critical mass, the frustration can lead a typically calm Taurus to bulldoze through the blockage in a sudden and ungraceful way. Sometimes this breakthrough is exactly what it needs, but more often, and especially when it comes to the body, it's a messy, disruptive process that could've come about in a more comfortable way. If you're chronically relying on this bulldozer effect to force you into change, it's a clue that you may be operating in an imbalanced Taurus retain-purge pattern.

To avoid this behavior loop in health or elsewhere, it's helpful for Taurus to befriend its natural tendency to resist. In consultation, when exploring resistance to change, I often hear Taurus people describe themselves as "lazy," but this has always proven to be inaccurate and unhelpful self-criticism. Resistance is important information for Taurus, and resisting resistance rarely uncovers your path forward. Instead, I encourage you to relate to your resistance, welcome it, feel its associated sensations in the body, and ask it what it needs. Beneath the resistance, you will often find that you feel unsupported, as though you can't trust your body or yourself, or perhaps that your concept of self-worth needs some attention. Although counterintuitive, treating resistance as a wise friend and attending to what's beneath it move Taurus gently forward in its health journey, dissolve obstacles, and prevent the bulldozer effect.

Other Planets in Taurus
Mercury in Taurus

Mercury in Taurus may need some extra help staying clear and alert. Brain food and strategically starting the day with protein and fat are nutritional priorities. Although Mercury tends to be sensitive to caffeine, this placement may benefit from stimulants in moderation. Longer breaks or gentle walks between meals may help improve this Mercury's cognitive function.

Mercury in Taurus is often a slow and deliberate mover. It's important to regularly break up slow, steady movement with a little bit of speed work, whether speed strength using weights or bodyweight quickness and agility.

Venus in Taurus

Venus in Taurus will likely face many opportunities to relate to pleasure and satiety in new, more embodied ways. Venus's soft, syrupy nature makes it more prone to insulin resistance and hypothyroidism as compared to other Taurus placements.

This Venus may be disinterested in exercise or may find that its tolerance for more intense exercise is low. Building lean mass through resistance training is often necessary to keep this Venus's body healthy, but movement that connects it with nature, beauty, or sensuality is nourishing for its soul.

Mars in Taurus

In both nutrition and exercise, Mars in Taurus is served best when it stays away from extremes and adopts a consistent, steady approach. But be aware that this Mars can also be very stubborn and may keep doing something long after it's stopped supporting them. Sluggish energy levels and stagnation are common.

Neck pain tends to plague Mars in Taurus. It's important to bring balance to the upper body by focusing on pulling movements (rows, pull-ups, deadlifts) as much as, or even more than, pushing movements. Longer warm-ups and punctuating strength work with quick movement bursts are wise too.

Jupiter in Taurus

Like Venus in Taurus, it's important for Jupiter in Taurus to explore themes of satiety and pleasure in eating. But it's also prone to accumulations, such as constipation, goiter, or insulin resistance. Be curious about how different carbohydrate-rich foods make you feel, both physically and mentally. If within financial means, keeping food simple but spending the extra money on high-quality, local ingredients may keep this Jupiter in bounds but still in touch with its opulent nature.

If it puts in the work, this Jupiter can get extremely strong. If it's not already doing it, weightlifting is highly recommended to support the metabolism.

Saturn in Taurus

Saturn in Taurus may shy away from indulging the senses and instead "indulge" fearful thoughts or attachment to strict eating patterns. This Saturn is prone to health ruts and may experience food fear and strong internal resistance to self-nourishment. Increased fiber consumption is very important in keeping this Saturn unstuck both physically and emotionally.

Like Mars in Taurus, this Saturn may experience chronic pain in the neck, occiput, and upper shoulders, possibly creating barriers to movement. However, if trained and fed properly, it can become a real powerhouse. Because it's prone to stagnation, mobility and flexibility should be regularly incorporated into its routine.

Uranus in Taurus

If Uranus in Taurus is aggravated, tooth pain or facial neuralgia may make getting enough nutrition very difficult, requiring a temporary reliance on soft foods. This Uranus may swing between extremes, whether in the thyroid, colon, or other Taurus area. If food contributes to this disruption, it may have some relation to Venus, including gluten, eggs, sugar, or dairy. In fitness, this Uranus may have a knack for explosive strength.

Neptune in Taurus

If Neptune in Taurus is a prominent chart player, it may contribute to symptoms of hypothyroidism. Neptune can allow things to "seep out," and there may be a lack of nutrients needed for proper thyroid function, including iodine, selenium, and zinc. Like Venus in Taurus, this Neptune may prefer movement that's sensual and beautiful.

Taurus Nourishment Checklist	Taurus Movement Checklist
Gesture: Pleasure	**Gesture:** Slow and Steady
✦ Allow satisfaction	✦ Get in nature
✦ Carb curiosity	✦ Increase NEAT
✦ High fiber, protein, and healthy fat	✦ Slow and controlled movement
✦ Support steady energy	✦ Strength focus
✦ Warm liquids	✦ Support metabolism

VIRGO

Virgo Anatomy

Ruled by speedy Mercury, Virgo is a busy type of Earth that's skilled in organizing, coordinating, separating, and assimilating. Virgo is a mutable sign, meaning it's not only Earth in motion but it excels at transforming material. In the body, we see Virgo transform earthen material from one form to another all the time via the miracle of digestion. This complex, multiorgan system is just the kind of thing that Virgo loves to orchestrate and where most of this sign's anatomy is found.

Mode	Ruling Planet
Mutable	Mercury

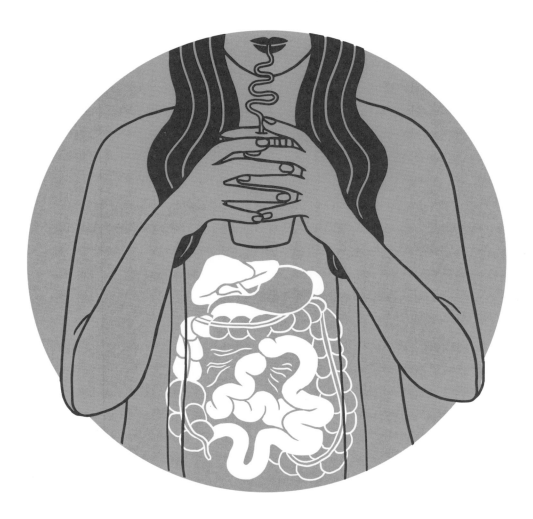

+ Diaphragm

+ Mesentery

+ Liver

+ Spleen

+ Pancreas (specifically its enzyme secreting function)

+ Small intestine

+ Enteric nervous system and gut-brain axis

+ Gastrointestinal immune system (with Pisces)

+ Sympathetic nervous system

+ Ascending colon

Virgo Nutrition

Gesture: Gut Feeling

The foundation of Virgo health is connection to gut feeling. Gut feeling is a deep inner knowing Virgo possesses that extends well beyond food. But within nutrition, the gut-brain axis is a vital piece. Keeping this axis of communication clear and supported equally on both ends is the focus of Virgo nutrition. Whether conscious of it or not, Virgo's first signs of nutritional imbalance are often cognitive. Virgo has a huge capacity to produce and perform, but because it's such a cerebral sign, it often doesn't realize it's gone too far until anxiety, nervousness, insomnia, and jumpiness are its daily experience. These symptoms indicate that one or both sides of the gut-brain axis need more strengthening and regularity. If this pattern goes unchecked for too long, classic digestive symptoms will become more obvious and pronounced.

Supporting Virgo Digestion

Because Virgo rules the abdomen, deep belly breathing is a fantastic way to begin meals. This practice helps Virgo enter a parasympathetic, rest-and-digest state—something that tends to be pretty challenging for this sign. Sit or lie comfortably and gently place one hand on your belly and one on your chest. Breathe in through your nose, allowing your belly to fill up like a balloon in all directions, even the back. Let the air out gently with an openmouthed sigh or through the nose—whatever feels most relaxing. Virgo often needs a bit more intentional settling than just taking three deep breaths. If you can, I encourage you to pause and do three minutes of belly breathing before serving your plate.

Virgo's ruler, Mercury, is always on the move, gathering information and making connections. This makes Virgo the intelligent and thorough sign that we love, but also tempts it to make simple things overly complex. Since a lot of Virgo's nutritional health is within the mind, you want to ensure that it's never nutritionally overwhelmed. Food is information too. When you approach food as information that can add to or subtract from a complex mental state, you may notice your food choices and food timing begin to shift. Perhaps eating smaller, more frequent meals feels supportive. Virgo commonly reports feeling uncomfortable with too much in the abdomen at one time. Large portions may feel as though they clog and confuse Virgo's delicate digestive process because there's suddenly so much to do and so much detail to break down. This may create both physical and mental stress and could result in poor absorption.

Another way to prevent nutritional overwhelm for Virgo is to keep meals simple, such as five ingredients or less. Again, this is to make sure you're giving the abdomen as much support as possible in separating, organizing, and breaking down the food it's given. Simple meals can also bring Virgo mental peace because the thought and preparation involved are less complicated. Simplifying food not only means reducing the number of ingredients but also focusing on basic flavors and textures. Virgo doesn't usually dislike spicy food, but such food may aggravate this sign and might feel best taken in smaller, infrequent doses. Ideally you want as few dietary extremes as possible entering a Virgo digestive system, whether via flavor, texture, amount, or timing.

Virgo thrives when food is warm, well cooked, and easy to digest. Although a plant-focused diet is a popular choice for this Earth sign, raw food is rarely Virgo supportive. This sign may like the idea of raw food, but when it comes to digesting it, the body and mind are often left with a large amount of stress. Create warm salads by lightly wilting, braising, or grilling greens and topping them with roasted vegetables and protein. If eating a raw salad, mince your greens finely with kitchen shears and use an acidic dressing that includes apple cider vinegar or fresh lemon juice to aid digestion. Liquid nutrition is another Virgo staple. By liquid nutrition I do *not* mean liquid diets or liquid fasts. Rather, this means warm, satisfying, and nutrient-dense liquid nutrition with adequate fat, protein, carbohydrates, and calories. When Virgo digestion is overwhelmed, softer foods can give it the complexity break it often craves. Virgo-friendly examples of liquid nutrition are broths, soups, stews, and elixirs. Cold juice and smoothies aren't recommended in large amounts for this sign, but you can make them more Virgo friendly by drinking them at room temperature, swapping frozen fruit for fresh, or using a steamed bland vegetable base, such as cauliflower.

Although all zodiac signs can suffer from food allergies, sensitivities, or intolerances, Virgo tends to be one of the most susceptible. Astrology *may* help identify which foods are problematic. For example, even though grains traditionally belong to Virgo, many Virgo people (and its sign pair, Pisces) are highly sensitive to gluten. You can find more information on astrology and food sensitivities in chapter 7. But where astrology is most helpful is in identifying which organs or body systems may need support while trying to heal sensitivities. It's also helpful in identifying any food stories, fears, or judgments that may be triggering a food reaction. When investigating the root of Virgo sensitivities, never rule out stress, but also talk to your health practitioner about the liver, bile production, and your ability to digest fat. Everyone needs healthy fat, but I've noticed in practice that Virgo tends to struggle with fat digestion a bit more frequently. As a Virgo person, if my GI symptoms are flared, I've found it helpful to eat my fattiest foods (like nut butter or avocado) as snacks, away from my main meals. Keep this in mind as you're navigating animal protein as well. Generally, Virgo digests light proteins such as chicken, turkey, pork, and fish with more ease.

Virgo Movement

Gesture: Awareness

Virgo energy is the lightest of all the Earth signs. When trained, it's agile but strong and makes challenging movements look easy. This type of grace and poise flowers out of well-developed body awareness. Just as gut feeling and the gut-brain axis are the roots of Virgo nutrition, awareness and the mind-muscle connection are the roots of Virgo movement. Enriching this connection not only requires intelligent routines but also the willingness to adapt them as the brain and body exchange subtle information. This often means slowing down, bringing your attention to the muscles being engaged, and regularly incorporating activation and corrective exercises for small muscle groups.

Head to clairegallagher.co/bodyastro for video examples of Virgo movements.

Virgo is a fan of mastering the basics. Although this sign lives for details, Virgo's love of complexity tends to be its biggest obstacle in movement. Virgo can be attracted to elaborate and busy exercise schedules, but if the focus is on the details instead of the foundation, it may never experience the benefits it's seeking. For Virgo, simple training is better medicine than complex training. Simple doesn't mean easy but rather an emphasis on efficiency and foundational movement patterns. No matter how you choose to move, go for quality over quantity and make your Virgo movement worthwhile by using mental presence, full range of motion, and great technique.

Supportive Virgo fitness is also repeatable, which requires giving yourself a dose of exercise you can handle. Just like large portions and complex flavors may leave a Virgo belly miserable, large and complex doses of exercise can leave a Virgo body overwhelmed. The waste and hormonal cascade produced by a monster session tend to keep Virgo tied up sorting and processing when it could be recovering for its next session. Frequent but timely and clearly directed sessions are typically the Virgo sweet spot.

Virgo Strength and Conditioning

In the world of strength and conditioning, Virgo reminds us to work on our bodyweight skill before we pile on the weight. A Virgo workout may be entirely bodyweight and often includes classic moves such as push-ups, pull-ups, chin-ups, and single-leg squat variations that many people find humbling. They're basic but certainly not easy, and they require a lot of practice. When we do bodyweight movements like these, it's easy to spot the holes in our strength. Compassionately identifying and then attending to our weaknesses are part of a well-rounded Virgo training program.

Another pillar of Virgo fitness is core development. This is a natural focus because of the core's role in sound movement patterns and because many of these muscles belong to Virgo. But please don't waste Virgo's time with endless sit-ups. Instead, the mutable nature of Virgo teaches us how to rotate, stabilize, and incorporate overhead movements that train the core by keeping it a part of the whole. Instead, try Turkish get-ups, overhead squats, front squats, and overhead walking lunges.

Virgo Running

Almost any type of running suits this Mercury-ruled sign, but Virgo may be drawn to the longer distances of half marathons, marathons, and ultramarathons. Endurance is a trait all the Earth signs share, but Virgo's light yet methodical energy translates well on the pavement. As a mutable sign, however, Virgo must incorporate variety to remain injury-free and keep its distance game strong. Make sure you're on a well-rounded running program that doesn't just focus on high mileage but leaves room for speed work, hill work, and cross-training as well. If you want to get super Virgo, hire a running coach and work on stride efficiency and foot strike.

Virgo Yoga

The emphasis of a Virgo yoga practice is alignment, posture, and core strength. Virgo may be drawn to traditions such as Iyengar, where the focus is on moving with precision and integrity. Although it's natural for Virgo to be on the go, it's also important to give the nervous system ample space to unwind. Be sure to supplement a dynamic practice with yin yoga, yoga nidra, restorative yoga, or other forms of deep relaxation. Include these more frequently at the New and Last Quarter Moons, but also use them to moderate the intensity of the Full Moon as needed. If you feel exhausted at the Full Moon, that's a whisper that you may have overextended yourself earlier in the month. Learn more about lunar cycle movement in chapter 2.

Other Virgo Sports and Classes

✦ Ballet

✦ Calisthenics

✦ Barre

✦ Core-focused classes

✦ Corrective exercise

✦ Gymnastics

✦ Pilates reformer

✦ Tumbling

Virgo Conditions

Instead of rock or soil, I tend to think of Virgo Earth as a tree, flower, or other plant. This type of Earth has a delicacy and flexibility to it, thanks to Virgo's mutable nature. Ironically, it's a lack of flexibility that gets most Virgo bodies and hearts in trouble. Physical and emotional imbalances tend to develop in this sign when it refuses to bend or adapt with life's changes. At best, Virgo is masterful, coordinated, and efficient, but at worst, it's debilitated and made rigid by details. When Virgo Earth is brittle, it often takes just one slightly amiss detail, enzyme, or function to put a whole system out of whack. Virgo conditions may include:

Anxiety or other sympathetic-dominant states

Celiac disease

Diverticulitis

Gas, bloating, alternating

constipation and diarrhea

Inflammatory bowel disease

Irritable bowel syndrome

Leaky gut syndrome (often reflexing to mood and cognition)

Liver sluggishness and overburden

Multiple food sensitivities, intolerances, or allergies

Small intestinal bacterial overgrowth (SIBO) and other gut microbiome imbalances

Although attractive to many Virgo-dominant people, counting calories, points, macronutrients, steps, or anything else is a practice best avoided. The more rigid Virgo is around food and movement, the more aggravated, neurotic, and tightly wound this sign becomes. In practice, I've found every instance of Virgo counting to be counterproductive to healing. Instead, it's often more beneficial for Virgo to release numbers and focus on reestablishing a relationship with their gut feeling. We've spoken about gut feeling in terms of the gut-brain axis and mind-muscle connection, but it's deeper than that. Gut feeling, also called "gut knowing" or "gut intelligence," is a deep self-trust and resolve to follow your own direction and wisdom. This is Virgo's birthright as the ruler of the abdominal organs and its connection with the rest of the body. When Virgo insists on counting and controlling, it's often at the expense of its own gut feeling and reveals a lack of trust in its own ability to guide and care for itself.

Another common Virgo practice is labeling foods as "good" or "bad." It's only natural for Virgo to sort, organize, and categorize, but when this line of thought becomes rigid, it creates a lot of suffering and increases the chances that Virgo will engage in disordered eating patterns. One of Virgo's talents is to create holistic systems. But when these systems become fixed and don't encourage constant connection with gut feeling, they can trap Virgo and sabotage its true essence, which is flexible and wise.

Virgo energy also tends to get swept up in new health trends. Again, this is usually a natural regression of long-term separation from Virgo's internal gut wisdom. Mature Virgo recognizes health trends as the mind-body stressors that they actually are. Virgo also knows that although it may love information, not all information applies to it. If Virgo is constantly on a new cleanse, detox, challenge, or protocol, it's distracting itself from what actually needs attention. In the psyche of Virgo, this is often a deep anxiety or fear that's prompting it to create the illusion of control.

Underlying most Virgo food and fitness issues is anxiety rooted in a belief that being in control equals safety. Hyper-controlling nutrition, exercise, or work is a very common knee-jerk response for Virgo when it's in this state. In many ways, this sign equates knowledge, data, and checking the boxes with safety. Mature Virgo understands that safety isn't found in numbers but in compassionate flexibility. This includes being flexible with your expectations of yourself and others and loosening up the black-and-white vocabulary you tend to use around wellness. For example, showing up for a workout doesn't make you "good" and missing a workout doesn't make you "bad." Befriending flexibility brings Virgo what it truly desires, which isn't control but peace.

Other Planets in Virgo
Mercury in Virgo

Mercury in Virgo often manifests as a very active mind that tends toward worry and nervousness. If food issues are present, instead of focusing on removing "problematic" foods, try focusing on removing problematic thoughts about food and managing stressful states at mealtimes. It's always wise to go easy on the caffeine if you have this placement.

Prioritize being completely present with movement instead of allowing your mind to run off. Until you get the hang of this, you may need to emphasize very engaging and mentally stimulating routines that demand your attention.

Venus in Virgo

Venus in Virgo's digestive system can be a bit cold and lax in its function and often needs more warm, liquid nutrition. Raw food is typically very hard on this Venus, and supplemental help is often needed to get the GI fired up before meals. Special attention should be given to regulating blood sugar.

This Venus might be very attracted to the softer expressions of Virgo exercise, such as yoga, Pilates, barre, or dance. Regardless of your movement interests, be sure to round out your practice by giving Virgo the rooting it needs in strength as well. It's also important not to hinge your self-worth on if you check or don't check off all the "wellness" boxes that mainstream culture serves us.

Mars in Virgo

Mars in Virgo may have more obvious, irritable, and inflammatory abdominal distress. But before running to an elimination diet, explore how stress or perfectionistic food thoughts and behaviors may be contributing to your GI experience. However, true food allergies are possible, with gluten, grains, and spicy food at the top of the list to explore. This Mars may need more protein and iron than other Virgo placements.

Be willing to frequently examine your often militant approach to fitness and nutrition. Mars in Virgo can become a tad obsessive and be more committed to a cause or idea than to its actual health. Be honest with yourself about any "wellness" practices that are actually creating stress, aggravation, and inflammation in your body and mind.

Jupiter in Virgo

Bloating and gas are the most common digestive complaints for Jupiter in Virgo. Jupiter is expansive, large, and rather uncomfortable in a detailed-oriented sign like Virgo. Jupiter and Virgo both rule the liver, and sometimes inadequate or congested liver function is at the root of gut problems.

This Jupiter can feel blocked by overly meticulous and rigid workout programs. Jupiter acts as a magnifying glass, and when in Virgo, it's common to not see the forest for the trees. Be sure that you're expanding upon the things that actually matter in your movement practice.

Saturn in Virgo

Saturn constricts and slows Virgo's body areas. For Saturn in Virgo, digestion tends to be cold, sluggish, weakened, and sensitive. Constipation-dominant IBS, poor breakdown, malabsorption, and nutrient deficiencies are possible. Food fear and restriction are often at the root of these conditions. This Saturn needs warm, well-cooked, easy-to-digest food that's fiber rich.

The Saturn in Virgo person is often very hard on themselves and tends to take an all-or-nothing approach in both fitness and nutrition. Healing your relationship to food and movement often involves reprogramming the black/white, yes/no, good/bad thinking patterns that Virgo is so prone to adopting. This placement may also indicate a compromised core that could be the root of other aches and pains in the body.

Uranus in Virgo

When agitated, Uranus in Virgo may express as anything acute in the gut. Sudden intestinal cramping, extreme and immediate changes in mood or cognition after meals, and reactive hypoglycemia are a few common examples. General health interests may be hit or miss as this Uranus vacillates between the Virgo perfectionist and the Virgo procrastinator.

Neptune in Virgo

Neptune can make the Virgo gut vulnerable to infection and invaders of all kinds, including candida, parasites, worms, or unwanted bacteria and viruses. Gut motion can be poor, allowing unwanted things to stick around longer. Neptune in Virgo's gastrointestinal immune system may be hyper- or hyporesponsive, sometimes resulting in food sensitivities. The mental state around food and fitness may be highly distorted or fear based.

Virgo Nourishment Checklist	Virgo Movement Checklist
Gesture: Gut feeling	**Gesture:** Awareness
+ Easy to digest	+ Alignment, form, full range of motion
+ Food as information	+ Bodyweight strength
+ Focus on feeling rather than numbers	+ Core development
+ Keep it simple	+ Master foundations
+ Well-cooked and warm food	+ Mind-muscle connection

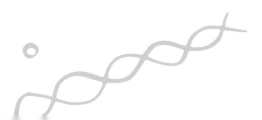

CAPRICORN

Capricorn Anatomy

Capricorn gives our flesh shape. If it's hard, durable, or acts as a framework or barrier, it probably belongs to this Earth sign. Capricorn is ruled by Saturn, who's obsessed with steadiness, righteousness, integrity, and the bones of things. Without Capricorn, we'd have nothing tangible through which to channel our life force. This sign provides a strong home for our ideas, dreams, and visions. In the body that translates to structure.

Mode	Ruling Planet
Cardinal	**Saturn**

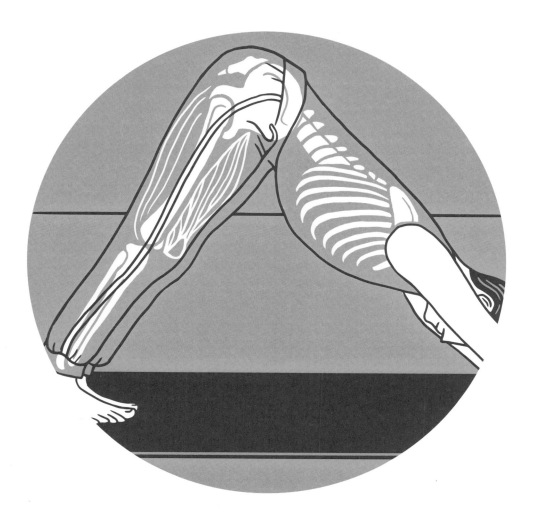

+ Bones (with Saturn)

+ Skin

+ Connective tissue

+ Joints, ligaments, and tendons (all joints, but especially the knees)

+ Teeth (with Aries, Taurus, and Saturn)

+ Nails and cuticles

+ Hamstrings

+ Gallbladder (with Saturn and Cancer)

+ Anterior pituitary gland (with Jupiter)

Capricorn Nutrition

Gesture: Sustenance

No matter the external weather, being born with a lot of Capricorn in your birth chart is like being born in cosmic winter. Regardless of which hemisphere you live in, traditional Capricorn foods are those we typically think of eating in cold weather: a stew with homemade bread, your grandmother's famous casserole, or the classic meat and potatoes. As the saying goes, Capricorn food sticks to your ribs. This type of food also tends to bring a feeling of comfort, a nod to Capricorn's nutritional partner, Cancer, and something every Saturn-ruled sign needs a bit more of. Because of its cold nature, Capricorn is naturally a meat-heavy sign, but meat-eater or not, all Capricorn bodies thrive when their plates are filled with warming preparations of hard squashes, root vegetables, and dark leafy greens. Capricorn food sustains and warms both your belly and your bones.

When feeding a Saturn-ruled sign such as Capricorn, you want to make sure that Saturn has all the nutrients it needs to stay healthy. Because of its association with karma, loss, limits, and a disproportionate amount of press about the Saturn return (see page 218), this planet often gets a bad reputation in popular astrology. Even in ancient astrology, Saturn was considered a malefic planet. There's truth to this, but without Saturn, we wouldn't have bodies, skeletons, skin, shelter, or anything tangible in our world. Instead of fearing Saturn, give it the materials to do its job properly. To adequately build and sustain us, Saturn and Capricorn need extra measures of foundational nutrients. When Saturn is malnourished, instead of building us up, it may feel like it's tearing us down or creating unwanted structure in the form of barriers and frustration. To meet the extra demands of Saturn, a priority of Capricorn nutrition is nutrient density. Nutrient-dense foods carry very high amounts of vitamins, minerals, and other beneficial content per serving size in comparison to other foods. Choose foods based on their nutrient content and ability to sustain you instead of worrying about their caloric content. Although every sign needs nutrient-dense foods, Capricorn typically requires an extra helping of the nutrients belonging to Saturn: protein, minerals, and vitamin C.

Sneaky Nutrients

It's important to pack as much nutrition as possible into each Capricorn bite. With just a few ingredient swaps and additions, you can incorporate more nutrients into your normal meal rotation. My personal favorite is to use bone broth to cook all grains and vegetables and as a substitute for water in almost any savory recipe. And you can increase the Capricorn nutritional content of warm drinks such as coffee, smoothies, or baked goods by adding collagen peptides or protein powder.

Wise Capricorn eats to strengthen its astrological anatomy, and this means eating both bone food and skin food. We can look at bone food a few ways: it physically maintains the skeleton, but it also maintains our energetic boundaries, personal strength, and integrity. These are all Capricorn life themes, and when using an astrological lens, they become doorways to greater Capricorn health. High-protein and mineral-rich foods are Capricorn staples because they energetically ground us, and when broken down, their constituents are used to maintain all of Capricorn's most important body areas. Feed your bones daily with dark green vegetables, egg yolks, fish, mineral-rich root vegetables, and nuts.

Vitamin C's functions in the body are endless, but its relationship to Saturn and Capricorn mainly comes from its role in collagen formation and antioxidant protection. A healthy Saturn—and therefore healthy Capricorn—says no to outside invaders by strengthening its first line of defense, the skin, and by managing free radical damage in the body. Eating for Capricorn skin health may require some curiosity around dairy and sugar. Capricorn needs a little sweetness in its life, but it occasionally affects the skin, joints, or gut. Capricorn often benefits from the bone nourishment found in high-quality dairy, but because it's partnered with Cancer, lactose intolerance is possible. Capricorn meals can be done on the cheap, but if you're going to splurge, dairy is the place. Focus on organic, local, full-fat dairy, and explore alternative and fermented sources. Goat and sheep cheese are often Capricorn friendly.

Lastly, barring any acute gallbladder or fat malabsorption issues (both frequent Capricorn complaints), ensuring you get enough high-quality saturated fat from coconut oil, eggs, fatty fish, grass-fed meat, and organic butter is a skin must. Capricorn people struggling with fat digestion may benefit from taking digestive bitters ten to fifteen minutes before meals.

Supporting Capricorn Digestion

Because it's ruled by Saturn, Capricorn is one of the coldest zodiac signs (Aquarius too). But digestion is a process that requires ample amounts of heat. You can help keep Capricorn's metabolism and GI humming steadily by sipping warm water throughout the day and refraining from drinking at meals (especially iced drinks!). Saturn also gives Capricorn its tireless work ethic. But for this sign to truly cleave nutrients from its food, it needs to separate work and meals. Digestion is enough work on its own. Leave work at your desk and reconnect with your Capricorn anatomy before meals by closing your eyes and lightly tapping on your knees.

Capricorn Movement

Gesture: Longevity

As the cosmic mountain goat, Capricorn's natural direction is to climb steadily upward. Its planetary ruler, Saturn, adds a density and heaviness to this climb, giving the imagery of walking uphill with a weighty pack. Natural Capricorn movement archetypes are hikers, trail runners, and winter mountain sport enthusiasts. But no matter if you're on the trail or in the gym, longevity is the backbone of Capricorn fitness. Wise Capricorn routines prepare this sign to go the distance and that means learning how to pace work properly, keep the effort sustainable, and support the body's ability to move for many decades to come.

We don't just cultivate longevity and endurance in how we move but also in how we think about movement. When working with a Capricorn, I want them to feel successful 100 percent of the time. Missing or shortening a workout, or simply modifying a movement, can often make them feel "unsuccessful" and knock them off course. To prevent this, I break Capricorn's program down into highly attainable chunks. I'll commonly limit beginners to one or two sessions per week at first, even if they come to me requesting five (a common Capricorn occurrence). I know that two is a more realistic number for them to maintain, which will give them the desired feeling of a steady climb without the shame cascade.

Because of the cold, dry, and often stiff nature of this sign, nutrition and recovery are just as important as Capricorn's actual workout program. Symbolic moisture must be inserted into the system, especially as Capricorn ages, via longer warm-ups and nonnegotiable mobility practice. Special attention should be given to the knees and the surrounding stabilizing muscles. Although not always natural for this forward-moving sign, developing the back of the body, specifically the hamstrings, to prevent imbalance and injury is also vital for Capricorn.

Capricorn Strength and Conditioning

In strength and conditioning, there are countless ways to enforce pacing, improve endurance, and mimic climbing energy by manipulating time, elevation, and other variables. Using high repetitions is a popular way to improve muscular endurance, but over the years, doing hundreds of repetitions each workout isn't very supportive of joint longevity or strength building. Instead of cranking out hundreds of reps, increase time under tension by using movement tempos or time prescriptions. It's a lot harder (and more efficient) to do eight very slow biceps curls at a challenging weight than twenty fast curls with super light dumbbells. We've talked about movement tempos in several other chapters, including Taurus (see page 144) and Aquarius (see page 128). Both Earth and fixed signs respond well to them.

In conditioning workouts, Capricorn challenges us to pace ourselves for the long haul. For example, completing a circuit of exercises without breaking until the end requires pacing. The goal isn't to finish as fast as possible but to complete each circuit roughly within the same amount of time. What this requires is sufficient rest, such as three minutes between circuits. You may think this sounds too long, but it's very intentional. Properly timed rest makes you more efficient and allows you to sustain hard work longer. Remember, the intention is endurance, which includes being able to continuously move through lengthy sets.

You can also simulate Capricorn's climbing energy in exercise selection. Stepping up, stepping down, crawling, and carrying weight over a distance support Capricorn. So is moving from a deficit or working at a decline or incline, as you might do with an incline bench press or decline push-ups. Deficit just means you're putting more space between your body and the floor. This makes an exercise more challenging and requires increased range of motion—another way to keep your joints healthy long term. You can do all sorts of movements from a deficit, but let's use the reverse lunge as an

Head to clairegallagher.co/bodyastro for video examples of Capricorn movements.

example. Create a small platform with a step or stack of weight plates (just a few inches will do). Stand on the platform and lunge back with your right leg, bringing your right knee to the floor. Because of the platform, your knee has to travel several inches farther to reach the ground, increasing the challenge and requiring more work.

Capricorn Running

Like the other Earth signs, Capricorn is often attracted to middle- or long-distance running, but it's also the Earth sign most likely to experience knee and other joint pain. Keep this in mind—not as something to fear but as a reminder that movement longevity is the larger goal. You probably want to keep running in the decades to come, and I want Capricorn to move well into its older years. This typically requires compromise and movement diversity. Try not to get stuck in a rut of only running. Movement ruts are one of the fastest ways to age a Capricorn body prematurely. To keep the bones and joints healthy, branch out and incorporate weight-bearing exercise, as well as plenty of Water sign movement to bring in some moisture and pliability. Check out the Cancer section (Capricorn's balancing sign) for some Water ideas.

Capricorn Yoga

Like Virgo, a Capricorn yoga practice has a strong focus on alignment, posture, and longer holds. As the bone ruler, Capricorn also has an increased need to focus on spine and joint health. Capricorn's body warms up slowly, so take your time and luxuriate in a long joint-circling sequence before a more vigorous practice. No need to put yourself in a 115-degree room, but a warm practice space will do this sign good. Again, the greater focus is longevity. It's never too early to start going to yoga classes that focus on healthy aging and joint care or even supplementing with tai chi or qi gong. Another Capricorn longevity tip is to bring yoga to work. A quick chair-and-desk sequence is the perfect break for this sign.

Other Capricorn Sports and Classes

+ Alpine skiing

+ Backpacking

+ Bouldering

+ Goat yoga

+ Hiking, trekking, mountaineering

+ Ice climbing

+ Mountain biking

+ Obstacle races

+ Rock climbing

+ Ultra-endurance events (bike, run, swim, walk)

+ Walking

Capricorn Conditions

When a Capricorn imbalance manifests, it's a clue to assess the foundation. They appear when the physical or emotional structures of the body have become too hard or too flimsy, or when the control mechanisms of the body are too overbearing or completely absent. In other areas of life, this may appear as difficulty establishing boundaries—whether yielding and passive or sclerotic and isolating—with yourself or others. Capricorn troubles force you to climb toward something better, but navigating them almost always requires hard work, investment, and patience. Capricorn conditions may manifest as:

Bone fractures and dislocations

Chronic muscle or joint pain and stiffness (arthritis, fibromyalgia)

Depression

Feeling cold

Fertility challenges

Gallstones, gallbladder inflammation, reduced bile flow, and other gallbladder imbalances

Hearing loss

Hypothalamic-pituitary-adrenal (HPA) axis dysfunction

Nutrient deficiencies and malabsorption

Osteopenia and osteoporosis

Scoliosis

Skin conditions of all kinds (acne, dryness, eczema, psoriasis, rash, sensitivity)

At the depths of many Capricorn food and movement issues is a fear of not being, doing, and having enough, or a fear of being inherently "wrong" or "bad." Capricorn will often choose suffering and hardship to prove that it's doing "enough" and doing it "right," but this attachment to blind climbing, and the fear of what may happen when it stops, often acts as a barrier to authentic success. To heal its relationship with food and movement, Capricorn often needs to redefine its concept of success and understand what motivates its constant climbing and what it's truly seeking by reaching the top. Deep, bone-level contentment and knowing that all is well, no matter where it is along the path, is often what this sign's heart and body need.

Longer work hours and scrolling to-do lists are common signs that Capricorn needs to pause and reset, but its goal orientation can also express as avoidance. This has nothing to do with "laziness" and everything to do with the mountainous expectations Capricorn tends to place on itself. The pressure to perform in one area is often so great that other parts of life, such as movement and nourishment, may go completely unattended. For some, this may manifest as viewing food as a waste of time or money, working through lunch breaks, or skipping meals altogether to get more done. Within movement, Capricorn may never begin an exercise program because it's afraid of disappointing itself and leaving its mountainous expectations unmet. Alternatively, Capricorn can become so obsessed and performative with food or fitness that other determinants of well-being (which are many!), like social, mental, or spiritual health, take a backseat.

Fear can also show up as long-term ruts or restriction. A Capricorn rut often looks like doing the same workout routine or eating the same thing for days, months, or years on end. Consistency is therapeutic for Capricorn to a degree, but when taken too far, the body is starved of the nutrient and movement diversity it needs to feel sustained. Ruts are often fear-based behaviors shielding Capricorn from the possibility of not meeting its own, or society's, expectations—no matter how skewed and unrealistic they are. Ruts keep Capricorn from having to maturely face and break free from its classic pass/fail approach to health and life. Restriction, although slightly different from ruts, is usually also rooted in fear. Like Virgo, it's often easier for Capricorn to count calories, steps, and macronutrients and remove entire food groups than it is to look underneath these behaviors and ask itself what it truly needs. Capricorn is wise to remember that the body carries the burden of all the work it endures and restricting its nourishment restricts its output.

Another sign to compassionately adjust Capricorn's food or movement approaches is symptoms signaling malnourishment or overwhelm. Joint pain, skin changes, feeling cold, and constipation are common signals that Capricorn can't process the load it has placed on itself. When left for too long, this can lead to an inversion of the classic Capricorn ambition and may show up as depression, listlessness, and feelings of purposelessness.

Other Planets in Capricorn

Mercury in Capricorn

For Mercury in Capricorn, if digestive issues are present, they're often exacerbated by high stress levels, eating on the go, or eating at a work desk. Prioritizing a small grounding ritual before meals is often more effective than dramatic dietary change for this placement.

This Mercury is prone to ambitious pacing and overdoing it. Be sure to create a workout routine that supports *your* long-term definition of success, which may mean focusing on sustainability and adjusting your expectations to be self-supportive. Joint pain is also common and, if present, often due to an aggravated or possibly impinged nerve.

Venus in Capricorn

For Venus in Capricorn, food issues typically show up as oily skin conditions with a hormonal root, possibly requiring increased consumption of healthy fat. This Venus often has trouble releasing waste products through the skin and may need to help the skin express via exercise, exfoliation, and other self-care practices.

Venus tends to soften the Capricorn body, making not only bone nutrition but also weight-bearing exercise high priorities. If joint pain is present, it may be due to weak supporting structures, and increasing muscular strength will often help.

Mars in Capricorn

For Mars in Capricorn, food reactivity may reflect in the skin as rash, dryness, flakiness, itchiness, or anything else that's red and inflammatory. Like Mercury, this Mars needs to manage stress around eating and avoid skipping or working through meals. Gallbladder inflammation is possible if high stress and poor eating habits are sustained long term. This Mars may need more protein than other Capricorn planets.

In movement, a Capricorn Mars may push through pain or other body signals to stop. It's prone to injury and inflammation of the joints, particularly the knees, and benefits from diversifying its movement practice and steering away from highly repetitive motion.

Jupiter in Capricorn

Jupiter in Capricorn may be prone to gallstones or fatty deposits in the liver. Although low-fat diets aren't a preferred long-term solution, this Jupiter may tolerate the least amount of dietary fat in comparison to other Capricorn planets. If digestive issues express in the skin, they tend to be oily in nature and, like Venus, need help expressing.

Buoyant Jupiter can sometimes feel constrained by Capricorn's classically serious approach to fitness. Release the long checklist of fitness "shoulds" and lighten up. Transform workouts into challenges and games or simply take them outdoors.

Saturn in Capricorn

Saturn in Capricorn is prone to weaker digestion, food ruts, restriction, and nutrient deficiencies. If food sensitivities or intolerances are present, the root problem is often a restrictive mindset or possibly a sleepy gallbladder and poor fat digestion. Digestive issues often show up as arthritic pain, lusterless skin and hair, or brittle nails. Since both Saturn and Capricorn rule the skeleton, bone nutrition and weight-bearing exercise are central to long-term health.

If fed and trained well, this Saturn has the potential to become very strong and resilient. But if malnourished, mistreated, or unwilling to question any harmful beliefs and behaviors around food and movement, the opposite tends to be true. Saturn is complex and can bring both strength and weakness to this sign—the outcome highly dependent on your previous choices and actions.

Uranus in Capricorn

For Uranus in Capricorn, extreme stress and a hyperproductivity mindset may contribute to acute digestive distress. Gallbladder attacks, stomach spasms, alternating constipation and diarrhea, acute skin reactions to food, or vomiting may appear. Uranus can send its shock waves across the zodiac to Capricorn's partner sign, Cancer, also creating spasm and disruption in the uterus. Uranus is prone to accidents and breaks, making bone strength and weight-bearing exercise extremely important.

Neptune in Capricorn

Neptune in Capricorn can weaken any of the body's boundaries, making them porous and leaky. A few examples are skin sensitivity, leaky gut syndrome, or even emotional enmeshment. Poor gallbladder function may contribute to digestive issues. A barrier to exercise may be joint pain or weakness. Neptune may need to supplement with bone- and joint-building vitamins and minerals such as vitamin D, calcium, and magnesium.

Capricorn Nourishment Checklist	Capricorn Movement Checklist
Gesture: Sustenance	**Gesture:** Longevity
✦ Bone building	✦ Frequent stretch breaks
✦ Nutrient dense	✦ Joint and spine care
✦ Saturn nutrient focus: protein, minerals, vitamin C	✦ Movement diversity
✦ Skin supporting	✦ Muscular and cardiovascular endurance
✦ Warming and grounding	✦ Sustainable pacing
	✦ Weight-bearing focus

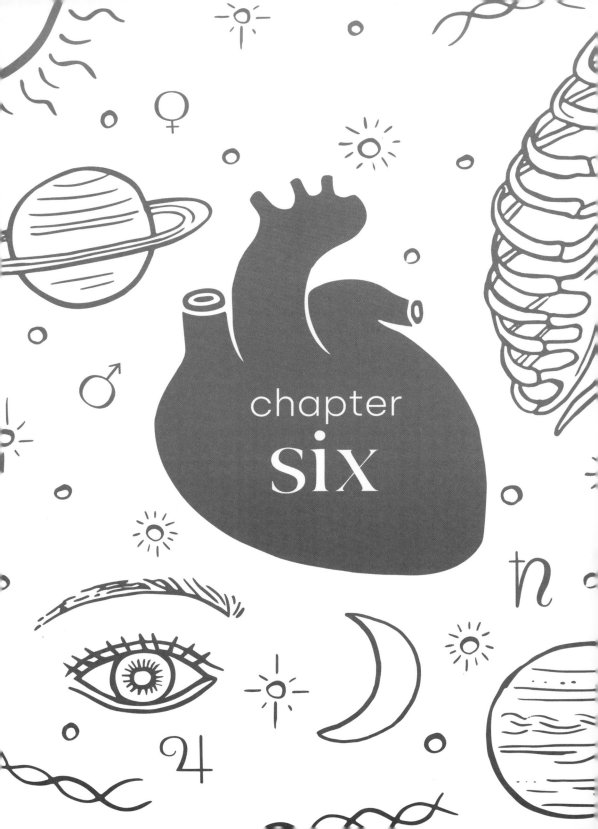

chapter
six

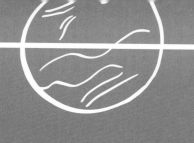
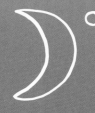

WATER BODIES

Signs: Cancer, Scorpio, Pisces

Qualities: Cold, Wet

Water may be the most misunderstood element in astrology. Descriptors such as sensitive, empathetic, and emotional are common, and while all these may be true, what tends to get left out in conversations about Water is power. Depending on its form, Water holds the power to sustain or end life. It can freeze or flood. It can cleanse or drown. It can quench thirst or carry disease. It's wise to let Water define itself, understanding that it may flow from one expression to the other or manifest several simultaneously.

By astrological quality, Water is cold and wet. Although Water comes in all different temperatures, in this context, cold describes how the energy in a Water body tends to move and behave. Cold slows, constricts, and moves inward or down. This may be reflected in the metabolism, circulation, or emotional terrain of a Water body, and it's our first clue in Water self-care. Nutrition, fitness, and supplementation for a Water body will often carry a warming effect to help offset its cold nature.

Wetness mixes, merges, and combines things. It's relational and receptive. Water also takes on the shape of its container. From these qualities arise common Water themes such as sensitivity, compassion, and depth of feeling. Although Air is considered the element of communication, Water is a transporter of unspoken messages that undulate through the body. Water signs must often learn which of these subtle messages are theirs to carry or theirs to let go. In the body, this element governs the many physical and energetic fluid highways, which include emotions, hormones, and lymph.

When cold and wet appear together, things can feel heavy. If you've ever jumped into a body of water fully clothed or been caught in a downpour, you know how drenched clothes hang on your body and stick to your skin. This is exactly what it's like when Water signs feel unwell. Too much dampness can create many issues in the physical, emotional, and energetic bodies, leaving the Water person feeing absolutely drowned or floating very far away from their intended shore.

The goal in all Water-body self-care is to ensure that Water runs clear and unobstructed. We want Water to be fully in tune, pure, and powerfully operational in its natural gifts of tenderness, compassion, intuition, and wisdom. But just as a river is held by land, Water is most potent and masterful when it's given some boundaries and direction. The nutrition, fitness, and self-care for this elemental type is designed not only to keep Water flowing but also to fully anchor its power.

Supporting Water Nutritionally

Remember that astrology and the body are dynamic, and you can have too much, too little, or neutral Water at any given time. Eating to support your Water may look different throughout your life. Whether it's days, months, or years apart, you may find yourself cycling through periods of eating to decrease or increase Water.

WATER NUTRITION

Decreasing Water	Increasing Water
Fermented vegetables (kimchi, sauerkraut)	Broths and soups
Fresh lemon and lime juice	Eggs
High-fat nuts (brazil nuts, macadamia nuts)	Fermented dairy
High-quality animal protein, oily fish, and other seafood	Grains (both whole and refined)
Low-carbohydrate vegetables (asparagus, broccoli, cauliflower, dark leafy greens, zucchini)	Natural sugars (fruit, honey, maple syrup)
	Root vegetables and hard squashes (all potatoes, butternut squash, delicata squash)
Low-glycemic sour fruits (berries, cherries, citrus)	Sea salt
	Seaweed
Warming spices (cinnamon, cumin, curry blends, garlic, ginger, turmeric)	Water-rich fruits (apples, berries, melons, oranges, peaches, tomatoes)
Well-cooked food	Water-rich vegetables (bell peppers, cabbage, celery, cucumbers, lettuce, mushrooms, zucchini)

Foods and Practices That May Disturb Water
Additives, preservatives, dyes, and synthetic ingredients
Excess amounts of high-glycemic foods
Excess alcohol
Excessively salty, spicy, greasy, or deep-fried foods
Excess amounts of raw food

CANCER

Cancer Anatomy

Cancer's body areas nourish or protect, or they do both. It's the mother of the body. In popular astrology, Cancer is often thought of as weak or weepy, but without Cancer we would be defenseless. Internally, Cancer soothes and distributes sustenance. Externally, Cancer fends off anything that threatens our safety. This sign covers all our basic needs: food, water, air, shelter, and love. Any body structure that holds nourishing substances or cradles vital organs typically belongs to Cancer.

Mode	Ruling Planet
Cardinal	**Moon**

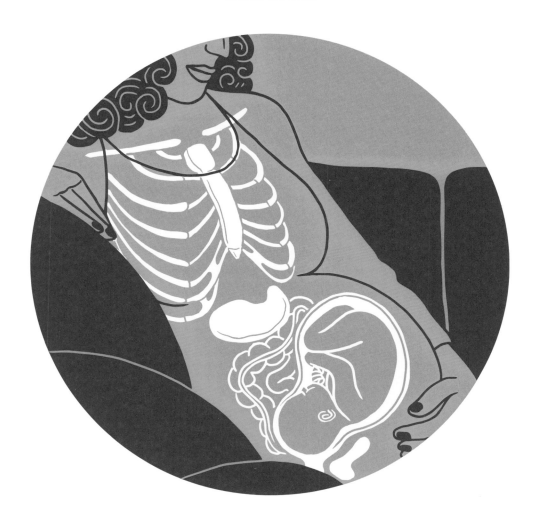

+ Meninges of the brain and spinal cord

+ Gums

+ Mucous membranes

+ Sinuses (with Taurus)

+ Lower esophagus

+ Chest, anterior shoulders (with Gemini), armpits

+ Breasts

+ Stomach

+ Gallbladder (with Saturn & Capricorn)

+ Sternum, ribs, intercostal muscles

+ Pericardium & pleura

+ Lower lobes of the lung

+ Diaphragm

+ Elbows

+ Flesh of the belly

+ Uterus (especially when pregnant)

+ Bladder (with Scorpio & Libra)

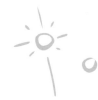

Cancer Nutrition

Gesture: Comfort

The primary nutritional focus for Cancer is to create a deep feeling of safety and trust in the body, no matter what state it's in. Embracing the body's and heart's vast and natural fluctuations is how Cancer creates a compassionate long-term relationship with itself, food, and anything else. What you're eating is certainly important, but how, where, and who you're eating with are often more pivotal. Cancer could have a "perfect diet" and still suffer greatly from digestive-related symptoms because of environmental or emotional stressors that haven't been tended to. Cancer benefits from doing as much mechanical and emotional work as possible outside of the digestive system. Addressing harmful food talk or thoughts and kindly tending to any emotions triggered by food are often more powerful than a complete nutritional overhaul.

Emotional Digestion

Cancer gets its deep-feeling nature from the Moon, its planetary ruler. Whether Cancer readily displays its emotions or keeps them hidden depends on the rest of the chart, but either way, "digesting" your emotions before digesting your food can be extremely supportive when healing any Cancer GI distress. Begin meals by placing one hand on your heart and one hand on your belly. Do an emotional scan and compassionately take note of anything you're carrying with you into the meal. Also, do an environment scan. Even if you're in a familiar space, peek over your shoulders and see and hear what's around you. This amplifies a feeling of security and settles the nervous system.

Comfort food is medicinal for Cancer, but this extends beyond the popular meaning. Aim to create comfort in the body and mind before, during, and after meals. This may mean eating at a pace and in a place that feels relaxed and easing into meals with a few deep breaths or a moment of gratitude. It may also mean tuning into your hunger and fullness signals and noticing if being too hungry or too full changes your experience of comfort. Comfort also means cultivating a nurturing food voice. This is a gentle voice that disarms the harsh judgments and emotional charge around food. Cancer is often very skilled and willing to use this food voice with others, but doesn't always extend the same softness and compassion to themselves. When eating or choosing what to eat, try speaking to yourself in the same tone you'd use with a child or best friend.

For some, comfort food may also mean physically "safe" foods—those Cancer knows it can eat without fear of feeling sick afterward. Cancer is one of the most food-reactive signs of the zodiac, so it's important for it to have a creative menu of allergen-free comfort food on hand. You can learn more about astrology and food sensitivities in chapter 7. If food reactivity is something you experience, take some time to remake your most cherished comfort-food dishes using Cancer-friendly substitutions. Because Cancer's natural qualities are cold and wet, foods that cause Cancer discomfort may also be energetically cold, wet, and sweet; they push Cancer into a state of Watery overflow. Be curious about dairy, eggs, and sugar. These foods are not "bad" for Cancer, but all three are cold and wet in quality and generate dampness or body fluids, which can feel aggravating when Water is already in excess. Sometimes high-quality, full-fat, and traditionally sour dairy can be therapeutic for Cancer, but if not, experiment with alternatives that create a creamy texture, such as coconut cream or blended cauliflower and avocado.

Developing an allergen-free menu may initially create the feeling of food safety that Cancer craves. But barring medical necessity, if the underlying emotional ties and food narratives remain unaddressed, there may come a point where this restriction simply becomes another emotional stressor. At this point, it's common for Cancer to begin reacting to formerly "safe" foods. Simply be aware of this potential pitfall and allow your healing process to fluctuate when it's ready to.

Cancer's tendency toward dampness also makes protecting the digestive fire a top priority. Pausing, breathing, and properly preparing to eat is the first way to stoke the flames, but this precious fire may also be protected by refraining from liquids before and during a meal. This can take some time to get used to, but it's worth it. If you must drink during a meal, stay away from ice and try your best to ensure that the beverage is hot or at least room temperature. You can also protect your digestive fire by being mindful of your consumption of raw and cold foods. High amounts of cold food often require energy to be "stolen" from other systems and shunted to the GI for help, resulting in fatigue, brain fog, and other symptoms after eating. You can also assist Cancer digestion with textures and food prep methods. Cancer digestive systems do especially well with mashes, puddings, purees, soups, and steamed food. Soft food assists Cancer by doing as much mechanical digestion outside of the stomach as possible. You can also make your proteins easier to digest by brining, marinating, and slow cooking your meats and by soaking grains and beans before cooking them.

Digestive dampness can also be moderated using flavor. Bitter and sour foods have a drying and somewhat astringent effect. Try adding something bitter to each meal—such as arugula, broccoli, Brussels sprouts, endive, or kale—to enhance digestion and help drain excess Water. Sour fruit such as berries, cherries, citrus, and green apples may also be useful. Baking fruit or making a compote doubles the Cancer nourishment.

Cancer Movement

Gesture: Intuitive

Cancer is ruled by the ever-changing Moon, which often puts the Cancer body and heart in a constant state of flux. This sign is highly attuned to changes in Moon phase, Moon sign, ocean tides, humidity, and body fluctuations from fluid balance and mood to the menstrual cycle. As you know by now, I want all signs to move with the Moon, but it seems to be doubly important for Cancer. Accepting and moving for your fluctuating body is one of the most supportive health decisions Cancer can make. This is often hard to do in popular fitness culture, where refrains such as "No pain, no gain" still take center stage.

Head to clairegallagher.co/bodyastro for video examples of Cancer movements.

But for Cancer, ease is gain and pain is pain. Sure, Cancer needs to move vigorously and sweat it out occasionally, but less is often more for this reflective sign. Use the lunar and/or menstrual cycle to wax and wane your workouts and always trust your movement intuition, even and especially when it goes against the popular "wellness" grain. For a deep dive into lunar fitness, head back to chapter 2.

Soft movement is a huge piece of Cancer fitness. I can't stress enough that Cancer's power comes from moderating yang. Too much yang—whether it's sunlight, sweat, spicy food, or stress—will eventually push a Cancer off course. Yes, Cancer needs to express its fierceness—after all, crabs have pinchers. But Cancer also needs ample space to contract and go inward—totally guilt-free. Cancer's workout schedule should be punctuated regularly with restorative movement. This includes yin yoga, yoga nidra, mobility, active recovery, and anything that incorporates deep or rhythmic breathing with long holds. Think blankets, cushions, foam rollers, bolsters, and low lighting.

A major theme of Cancer well-being is cultivating safety, which is relevant in exercise too. An uncomfortable environment is one of the most common Cancer movement barriers. Many Cancer-dominant people prefer to work out at home. It's comfortable and you don't feel vulnerable or on display. You can get a lot done with just a yoga mat, a pair of dumbbells, and a kettlebell. Plus, it'll all fit under your bed. But if you don't have the space or funds to create a home gym, do some gym research. Find the times that are least crowded and when the trainers aren't walking the floor. Use these times to get acquainted with the equipment and the free weights at your own pace without feeling exposed. Do whatever you need to feel comfortable in your workout. For my Venus in Cancer, that means an oversized black hoodie, hat on, headphones in, and exoskeleton vibes high.

Speaking of safety, Cancer is quick to defend and has a fighting streak that may surprise you. Some unexpected athletic archetypes of Cancer are found in combat sports: boxing, wrestling, karate, mixed martial arts, and jujitsu, to name a few. The common denominator in these athletes is the use of their "exoskeleton" to protect something or someone. Whether you discover you have a deep interest in self-defense or find you simply enjoy dropping in for a kickboxing class once per week, these movement modalities mature, soothe, and strengthen Cancer on all planes.

Cancer Strength and Conditioning

In its approach to strength and conditioning, Cancer teaches us to bring more fluidity into the weight room. When I'm creating a Cancer strength workout, I like to blend harder and softer modalities together and end up with a fun mash-up of bodyweight flow, weighted flow, mobility, punching, and kicking. By flow, I mean graceful movements done seamlessly, almost as though you're dancing with the weight. When working with Cancer, I'll often punctuate heavy barbell sets with yogic-inspired flow sequences or even kickboxing intervals. Strength-flow sessions leave me feeling resilient but flexible—the perfect Cancer combo. We see this theme in Pisces strength too.

To keep Cancer's anatomy strong, also be sure to focus on upper body strength. Boxing-inspired workouts are naturally upper-body focused, but don't forget about push-ups, plank variations, bench presses, and other exercises targeting the chest and anterior shoulders. These muscles belong to Cancer, and strengthening them can energetically assist you in drawing proper boundaries in your life—a necessary Cancer skill.

But perhaps more important than the workout contents is your commitment to self-love and awareness as you move. I'm all about having an organized program, but have you ever done an intuitive lifting session? It's

Cancer magic. Being able to lift weights intuitively requires a little prior experience and knowledge, but once you have a foundation, you can head to the gym (or home gym) with a training intention and just flow from movement to movement as your body guides you. I do intuitive routines during the New or late waning Moon, when I'm mentally fatigued, or menstruating—basically anytime I want to move but don't have the energy for a full workout.

Cancer Running

Although any sign can love or despise running, this type of forward churning motion isn't all that natural for Cancer. Cancer is more of a tide pool or bubble bath, and its energy tends to flow down and in toward stillness. Also, consider how a crab travels laterally instead of front to back. Cancer often takes an indirect route. There are always astrological exceptions, but Cancer running tends to either be unhurried or has ample space to fluctuate speed or intensity mid run. A fartlek run is a great Water running tool. Swedish for "speed play," a fartlek run is like an intuitive interval session—no clock required. In a fartlek run, you interrupt a moderate jog (or walk) with faster running. Use trees or other markers to keep your pace. For example, run hard until you reach the tree at the corner and then continue your moderate jog until the next tree or mailbox and so on.

Cancer Yoga

A Cancer yoga practice is about creating comfort and restoration. No matter what type of flow you choose, using props such as bolsters, cushions, blankets, straps, blocks, and movement modifications is highly encouraged. You want to give the body whatever it needs to feel secure. Intuitive yoga sessions are also very Cancerian. Light some candles, get on the mat, and allow your body to wave and undulate in whatever way it wants. Practicing Moon Salutations (*chandra namaskar*) is also very supportive for this sign. Instructions for this symmetrical and circular flow can be easily found online. It's the perfect balance to the frequently used and very heating Sun Salutations.

I've talked a lot about Cancer becoming imbalanced when yang, or heat, is in excess, but the flip side is true too. If you're experiencing Cancer imbalance symptoms and you only do yin forms of yoga, you may be experiencing an overwhelming amount of Water, and you could benefit from a couple more vigorous sessions during the week.

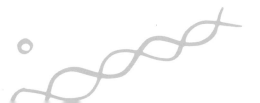

Other Cancer Sports and Classes

- ✦ All home workout systems
- ✦ Belly dancing
- ✦ Boating
- ✦ Bodysurfing
- ✦ Fishing
- ✦ Ground-based workouts, such as Animal Flow
- ✦ Kickboxing
- ✦ Martial arts
- ✦ Self-defense classes
- ✦ Skimboarding
- ✦ Snorkeling
- ✦ Spelunking
- ✦ Tubing
- ✦ Water aerobics

Cancer Conditions

Most Cancer conditions arise when there's a resistance to or rejection of fluctuation and a demand that the heart, mind, or body be other than it is in the present moment. If Cancer can truly lean on the Moon's promise that it will always find fullness again, it'll create an amazing home in the wise cyclicality of the body. When a Cancer soul feels unsafe or malnourished or if its emotional needs are unmet, the body will respond with a mirroring symptom. No matter where Cancer imbalances manifest, the common root among all of them is often emotional. When an emotional root or trigger is identified and attended to, the body often heals in tandem. Cancer conditions may manifest as:

Asthma

Breast swelling, tenderness, and cysts

Chronic fatigue with a digestive, emotional, or trauma-related root

Digestive discomfort: poor appetite, nausea, vomiting, stomachache, trouble swallowing, slow gastric emptying, too little or too much stomach acid, gas, bloating, diarrhea, prone to food poisoning

Dysbiosis

Eating disorders

Food fear and neuroses

Food sensitivities, allergies, and intolerances

Fungal overgrowth (*Candida albicans*)

Menstrual irregularities and hormonal imbalances

Sinus and respiratory infections

Water retention, swelling, edema

I've heard many Cancers say they can't trust themselves with their own food and movement needs. The exact reasons vary, but a common story is that they feel consistently sabotaged by large emotional and physical fluctuations. Although these fluctuations are very real, the belief that they exist to derail your health is untrue. The Moon is the planet of bodily nourishment, and as the Moon-ruled sign, Cancer's birthright is to be highly attuned to its nourishment instincts. Cancer's emotional fluctuations are a pivotal part of its health guidance system. When Cancer views emotional fluctuations as informants instead of irritants, it can create the space and neutrality it needs to learn from strong emotions without getting swept away by them. After practicing this for a while, you will become open to the possibility that sometimes moods don't mean anything and it's okay to let them be without attaching meaning to them. When Cancer befriends its fluctuating nature, it builds self-trust, which allows intuitive approaches to eating and exercising to work very well. But it's important for Cancer to understand that emotions and intuition aren't the same.

Cancer often self-identifies as an emotional eater. Unfortunately, this phrase carries a lot of judgment, and because of that, I don't love to use it. However, it is common for Cancer to use both food and movement as emotional processing tools. This is normal and healthy for Cancer until they become emotional override tools. Keep in mind that "emotional" eating or exercising may also include using diet tools or health food and exercise obsession to distract yourself from a difficult situation or emotion. Eating will never be emotionless for Cancer; nor should it be. Instead, healthy eating for this sign involves being a conscious participant in the emotions and stories surrounding food. This requires a willingness to look at emotions with compassion and clarity, and asking if food (or movement) is the best response. Developing emotional processing and coping tools beyond food and movement is very worthwhile for Cancer.

If you find yourself eating in response to a difficult emotion when you're not physically hungry, that's okay. Just recognize it's often a signal that your needs are unmet elsewhere. When a strong feeling arises, before reaching for food or movement, pause and ask if that's what the feeling needs. For example, "I feel X. What's the true need beneath this feeling? Will this need be met by eating Y or by doing Z workout?" The power of this practice isn't in what you eat or choose to do next, but in the commitment to turning inward, acquainting yourself with your needs, and giving yourself the space and opportunity to meet them.

Other Planets in Cancer
Mercury in Cancer

Mercury in Cancer carries a deep connection between the stomach and stress. Bloating, nausea, or appetite and bowel changes with nerves are all common. It's like a feedback loop—when thoughts are difficult, digestion is difficult; when digestion is difficult, thoughts are difficult. Food sensitivities tend to show up as slowed nervous system reactions and foggy cognition.

Like the digestive feedback loop, mood impacts this Mercury's desire to move, but movement heavily impacts mood. All exercise—particularly slow, meditative modalities—helps this Mercury process and gain clarity.

Venus in Cancer

For Venus in Cancer, food and digestive issues tend to express as sadness, defensiveness, or reclusiveness. The connection between the menstrual cycle and digestive health is also highlighted. This Venus may experience large water fluctuations in the middle of the body. There may not be adequate stomach organ tone, acid, or digestive enzymes, making it more prone to dysbiosis and GI infections.

This Venus may be very moody, and exercise is often used as a spirit lifter and emotional processing tool. Although this is a sensitive and tender Venus, the exercise intensity typically needs to match the intensity of whatever it's feeling.

Mars in Cancer

For Mars in Cancer, food reactions tend to be fast and intense with acute pain, irritability, and possible vomiting. There are often issues with stomach acid, whether too much or too little. It's more likely for Cancer to have deficient stomach acid, although the result may feel hot and fiery like reflux. Spicy food often gives this placement grief.

Prone to anger, whether repressed or overtly expressed, this Mars often benefits from a physical outlet for any rage it's experiencing. Combat sports are particularly therapeutic for this placement, but anything that allows it to move excess heat, engage with power, make noise, and emote will do.

Jupiter in Cancer

Jupiter in Cancer is prone to accumulating water as the lunar or menstrual cycle fluctuates. Water retention, swelling, edema, and distention are all possibilities. The liver may also be sluggish, and moderating foods that generate dampness may be helpful at times. Leaner proteins, low-carb vegetables, and low-glycemic fruit may support this Jupiter when feeling imbalanced.

Jupiter in Cancer may feel more at home with slow, fluid movement modalities. However, for long-term health, it may be important to moderate excess Water by generating some heat and working up a sweat. This Jupiter may need help improving its metabolic rate with a combination of strength and cardiovascular work.

Saturn in Cancer

Saturn in Cancer's digestive system tends to be somewhat repressed and highly sensitive. The stomach gets full quickly, and the appetite is often poor and tends to disappear with emotional upheaval. Digestive secretions are often inadequate and protein digestion tends to be difficult, resulting in poor nutrient assimilation and undigested food in the stool.

This Saturn may have a lot of restriction in the center of the body, manifesting as poor mobility in the thoracic spine, weak core, difficult breathing during exercise, or even feeling unsafe. There may be some exercise insecurity with this placement. Creating a comfortable movement environment can help warm and open up this Saturn both physically and emotionally.

Uranus in Cancer

When agitated, Uranus in Cancer can experience all types of digestive reversal like vomiting, belching, hiccups, nausea, acute stomach pains, and stomach acid irregularities. Severe uterine cramps and menstrual irregularities are also possible. Sometimes this Uranus can reject nourishment, whether through disordered eating or a psychological aversion to self-care.

Neptune in Cancer

Neptune in Cancer may lack sufficient gastric secretions, increasing susceptibility to weak digestion or GI infections. This Neptune may also experience an excess amount of dampness in the body, possibly adding to a global sense of fatigue and sensitivity. Neptune in Cancer may be prone to mold toxicity and fungal infections and find it's aggravated by raw and cold food, commercial dairy, eggs, and excess carbohydrate or sugar consumption. The cardiovascular system often needs targeted strengthening.

Cancer Nourishment Checklist	Cancer Movement Checklist
Gesture: Comfort	**Gesture:** Intuitive
✦ Calm eating environment	✦ Comfy movement space
✦ Comfort food	✦ Moderate yang
✦ Digest your emotions	✦ Move with the Moon
✦ Nurturing food voice	✦ Space to fluctuate
✦ Protect digestive fire	✦ Strength-flow combos
✦ Soft, warm food	

SCORPIO

Scorpio Anatomy

Scorpio rules the body systems that undulate beneath the surface of casual conversation. They're usually unseen, unheard, and unfortunately often associated with shame. But the Scorpio body propels our world, infuses it with power. Without it, life would cease to exist. Scorpio has an interesting three-pronged physiological purpose in the body. It concentrates, expels, and transforms. It distills energy, waste, by-products, and experiences until they're in a form that can exit the body safely. If this transformational function gets stuck, we're at risk of contamination. All organs of elimination, or emunctories, belong to Scorpio. The primary emunctories are the intestines, skin, kidneys, bladder, and lungs—I like to also include the emotions. Many of these tissues are shared with other signs, but when they're eliminating, they use Scorpio's channels.

Mode	Ruling Planets
Fixed	Mars (traditional)
	Pluto (modern)

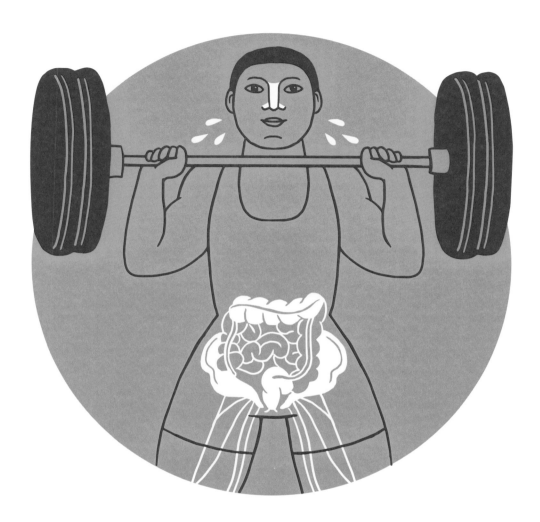

+ Sweat glands

+ Nose

+ Reproductive function & organs: uterus, ovaries, prostate, testes, genitals

+ Ureters, urethra, bladder

+ Colon, rectum, anus

+ Sacrum, coccyx

+ Groin and inner thigh muscles

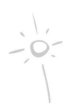

Scorpio Nutrition
Gesture: Transformation

The goal of Scorpio nutrition is to assist the body in transforming food into energy and then eliminating waste easily and efficiently. Intestinal health is a top priority, making regulating bowel habits, consuming fiber, and incorporating pre- and probiotic foods focal points for this sign. Scorpio nutrition also caters to its martial nature. Being Mars-ruled makes Scorpio the hottest Water sign and a rather fast metabolizer. It tends to thrive on protein and food timing that keeps it feeling energized and ready for action.

Scorpio and its partner sign, Taurus, need the most fiber. But Scorpio's intestinal picture can be complex. One type of fiber may cause a lot of aggravation, while another brings relief. Soluble fiber forms a gel in the intestines, gives stool some shape, and slows things down. Insoluble fiber doesn't form a gel and stimulates the gut wall mechanically, giving fiber its laxative effect. Insoluble fiber is usually a safe choice for constipation, but if you're dealing with chronic soft stools, eating a plate of roughage, no matter how "healthy" it seems, may trigger an inflammatory response in your body. Although both ends of the spectrum show up in Scorpio, it's more common to see chronic diarrhea or mixed pictures in this sign, and focusing on viscous soluble fiber is usually necessary. There's a blend of both fibers in most foods, but if you're dealing with a severe intestinal issue, you may want to pay close attention to your soluble versus insoluble fiber intake. Always increase your fiber consumption gradually and drink tons of water to reduce the chances of unwanted gastrointestinal distress.

Know Your Fibers

If you need more soluble fiber, stock up on apples, avocado, banana, beans, berries, chia seed (in liquid), citrus, flaxseed meal, oatmeal, parsnips, plantain, psyllium husk, sweet potato, taro root, turnips, white rice, winter squash, yams, and yuca root (also called cassava, tapioca, manioc).

If you need more insoluble fiber, stock up on alliums (garlic, leeks, onions), bell peppers, celery, coconut (flakes, flour), cruciferous vegetables (broccoli, Brussels sprouts, cabbage, cauliflower), whole grains (amaranth, brown rice, quinoa), greens (arugula, collards, kale, lettuce, spinach), nuts and seeds (almonds, walnuts), and radishes.

Scorpio tip: Make insoluble fiber foods easier to digest. They're better tolerated when fully cooked, blended, mashed, diced, de-stemmed, peeled, or fermented.

~~~~~~

Scorpio can also suffer from masked digestive symptoms that seem unrelated and show up elsewhere in the body as mood swings, pain, anxiety, skin conditions, or recurring urinary tract infections (UTIs) and yeast infections. Colonizing the gut with beneficial bacteria is a Scorpio focus because the benefits extend beyond the belly and trickle into many other body systems, including the skin, emotions, cognition, and hormones. Before reaching for a pre- or probiotic supplement, start with food. Prebiotic foods *feed* beneficial bacteria and include asparagus, beans, garlic, legumes, onions, and many other vegetables. Probiotic foods—such as kimchi, sauerkraut, other fermented vegetables, kefir, and yogurt—*contain* beneficial bacteria. The friendly microbes in these foods fight invaders, eat up the damaging toxins they produce, manufacture vitamins and short-chain fatty acids, and help us convert nutrients into forms our bodies can use. Like fiber, increase the consumption of fermented foods slowly, especially if you're dealing with GI symptoms. Treat them as side dishes or condiments. Even a couple of tablespoons can be very medicinal.

Hormone imbalances are such a prevalent Scorpio complaint that they need to be considered in daily nutrition. When Scorpio presents with a hormone imbalance, whether high or low, the root issue is often in the gut, not the reproductive organs. Let's take estrogen, for example. After leaving the liver, the gut is the primary way estrogen exits the body. Microbes in the gut produce an enzyme that can reactivate estrogen, allowing it to reenter circulation. When there's a gut imbalance, this enzyme's activity changes and estrogen levels may become too high or too low. Bottom line: the gut-hormone relationship is pivotal for Scorpio, and healing the microbiome typically has a direct and positive impact on other Scorpio complaints.

Scorpio's colon can be heavily burdened and often needs assistance from the rest of the body. Beyond improving intestinal health, Scorpio needs to make sure that the rest of its detox organs are open and working well. Although Scorpio finds them intriguing, dramatic detoxes and cleanses are *not* part of sustainable Scorpio nutrition and tend to do more harm than good. Instead, it's best to create an entire emunctory-supporting lifestyle. Your body is detoxing all the time. Scorpio just needs to enhance what the body is already doing. Regular exercise, mature emotional expression, a vegetable-heavy menu, lots of water, being mindful of your sugar and alcohol intake, and removing toxic products from your cleaning and beauty regimen are all ways to support your daily detox processes.

Scorpio Movement

Gesture: Power

Scorpio is ruled by the red-hot fire of Mars and driven by Pluto, the power-hungry god of the underworld. It's one of the strongest signs of the zodiac and most of its exercise modalities are very passionate and intense. Whether experienced in body or mind, most Scorpio issues arise from a power imbalance. This sign may feel like it swings between implosion and explosion. Conscious movement can integrate this jagged polarity and teach Scorpio how to use its power maturely. If you want to wield Scorpio power with wisdom, you must practice. The goal of Scorpio fitness is not foolish exhaustion. Rather, the goal is to become a master of transformation. From an exercise perspective, this means flirting with your personal threshold, where the veil is thin, but having enough control to ride the wave, not crash past it. Intensity is a skill you must practice, and over time your threshold will increase.

But there's another side to Scorpio movement that's just as powerful, but a bit subtler in its expression. The trademarks of these modalities are typically sensuality, depth, and undulation, and they're often performed in classes and environments that create an intense emotional response via lighting and music. A few common examples are pole dancing, primal movement, and burlesque dance. It's important for Scorpio-dominant people to have a foot in both realms—intensity and power complemented and balanced by their choice of moody and dramatic self-expression.

Scorpio Strength and Conditioning

Peak performance and power are the foundations of Scorpio strength and conditioning. We encounter these things in powerlifting, Olympic weightlifting, and metabolic conditioning workouts. Metabolic conditioning is exactly what it sounds like—training your metabolism to work like a well-oiled machine. We use this type of training to teach our metabolism (how we deliver and use energy for activities) to work at maximum efficiency. When most people hear metabolic conditioning, they think this means to crush themselves until they're utterly exhausted. But this common Scorpio pitfall doesn't benefit our metabolism in any way. When we're working at true peak, we can only sustain it for a limited amount of time. Only a small dose is needed to create a trans-formational stimulus.

Crafting an efficient metabolism requires strategy. Don't do high-intensity workouts every day and give your conditioning workouts limits so that you're flirting with your threshold but not constantly in the red zone. When we strategically use limits or controls in our conditioning workouts, we can meet intensity again and again and again. This keeps our session potent and primes our metabolism to be red-hot and efficient. Otherwise, we're just going through the motions in a prefatigued state, and although everything feels hard, the intensity has been slashed in half. Supercharge your conditioning sessions by keeping movements simple, lifting at submaximal loads, and adding strategic rest. To keep yourself from moving too fast, you could incorporate isometric exercises, use cyclical cardio intervals, or just aim to stay at 85 percent effort throughout. For most people, total conditioning work time (not including extended rest periods, warm-up, or cooldown) should range from about five to twenty minutes.

Head to clairegallagher.co/bodyastro for video examples of Scorpio movements.

Scorpio Running

Because Scorpio and Aries are both ruled by Mars, they have a similar approach to running. Running sprints at max speed is certainly one way to do a Scorpio run. But because it's a fixed Water sign, Scorpio tends to extend its intensity a little bit longer. Instead of working at 100 percent like we might do in an Aries sprint, I want Scorpio to do what I call "threshold running." This approach has lots of names in the running world, but they all involve the runner flirting with their maximum but not pushing past it. Done over time, this increases their maximum, making them faster and more powerful. Here's a basic example: After a thorough warm-up, run at 90 percent effort for two minutes. Walk for two minutes to recover. Repeat for five to eight sets, or as many times as feels challenging. Once you start having trouble recovering within two minutes, that's a good clue to stop for the day. You can do this type of run anywhere you choose, but I suggest a track where it's easy to visualize distance. Aim to cover the same amount of distance during every two-minute running interval.

Scorpio Yoga

A Scorpio yoga experience emulates this sign's trademark intensity in mood or body, or both. The practice tends to support catharsis or awaken power. Remember from the nutrition section that Scorpio needs to release, and this translates into yoga as well. This may be encouraged by lighting and music, temperature, intense sequences that promote sweating, or long holds with breathwork. All of these give opportunities for body memory, emotion, or even trauma to be transformed. A Scorpio yoga practice undulates and churns, bringing whatever is lurking at the watery bottom up to the top. Pelvic instability or congestion is a common Scorpio issue, so also include regular groin and hip mobility in your routine.

Other Scorpio Sports and Classes

+ Pole dancing

+ Burlesque dance

+ Primal movement

+ Buti yoga

+ Tantra yoga

+ Whitewater rafting and kayaking

+ Scuba diving

+ Survival training

+ CrossFit

+ Powerlifting

+ Olympic weightlifting

+ Hockey

+ Snowboarding

+ Rugby

Scorpio Conditions

Scorpio is a fixed sign, which means part of its job is to consolidate, condense, and hold on to things. Scorpio imbalances usually occur when there's too much retention and too little release, or too much release and too little retention. Either way, the transformative process that's so vital to Scorpio's well-being remains incomplete. Whether it's being blocked emotionally or impeded physically, avoiding transformation is where Scorpio imbalances tend to begin. Most, if not all, Scorpio conditions are rooted in the organs of the lower abdomen. When toxicity increases to a critical point there and isn't transformed, it begins to show up elsewhere in the body or in the emotional state. Symptoms on the surface aren't always what they seem and are rarely isolated events. Scorpio wants you to dig. When searching for the source, the best place to start is the lower gastrointestinal system or the genitourinary system. Scorpio conditions may manifest as:

Acne, boils, cysts

Bladder or urinary tract infections and incontinence

Body odor and excessive sweating

Chronic nasal congestion or runny nose

Diarrhea; constipation; alternating constipation and diarrhea; incontinence; bowel movements accompanied by pain, strain, or bleeding; hemorrhoids; irritable bowel syndrome (IBS); inflammatory bowel disease (IBD); bowel toxicity; parasites; bacterial infection or overgrowth; viral infection; yeast overgrowth; worms

Groin pulls and injury or weakness of inner thighs

Interstitial cystitis

Odd discharges anywhere in the body

Ovarian cysts, uterine fibroids, endometriosis, polycystic ovary syndrome (PCOS), premenstrual syndrome (PMS), premenstrual dysphoric disorder (PMDD), irregular menstrual cycles

Pelvic pain

Rage, obsession, fits, depression

Sacroiliac joint issues

Sexually transmitted infections

Vaginal yeast infections

Scorpio is the master of cycles and its job is to transform energy from one form to another. If any cycle in Scorpio's life, body, or heart gets stuck, it's a sign to reset. We see Scorpio's cyclical nature in birth and death, but this sign helps us transition in all contexts—sleep/wake, ingest/excrete, create/destroy, ovulate/bleed, anabolize/catabolize. Healthy Scorpio understands that all things slip away and are made new again. Suffering arises when this transformation is blocked or occurs too quickly, becoming a painful ride of dramatic outbursts, destruction, and self-sabotage. Part of Scorpio's health journey is learning how to ride within cycles and allow them to happen, instead of forcing or rejecting them.

Scorpio's major body cycles are excreting, emoting, repairing, and reproducing. Any large changes in bowel movements, urination, menstruation, or sexual function are clues that Scorpio's transformative process needs smoothing out. Like all Water signs, a lot of physical healing can occur on the spiritual-emotional plane. Scorpio's physical imbalances certainly need physical medicine, but learning to support transformation on a spiritual level can enhance and make this healing more complete. Become a student of transformational cycles in low-stakes situations—the birth and death of a season, the lunar month, or a single day or the rise and fall of your mood and energy levels. Notice any resistance or physical and mental anguish that arises as these changes occur. Attend to them maturely and ask how you can support the process. When we make room for these daily births and deaths, we increase our skill level in renewing and regenerating, and we learn how to care for ourselves in larger transitional contexts.

In the realm of nutrition, stuck cycles may appear as states of food fixation, control, or self-punishment. It's common for Scorpio to engage in disordered eating behaviors, which can take many forms. Severe caloric restriction, improper use of fasting, frequent use of cleanses, mono diets, and excluding entire macronutrients or food groups are just a few examples. In all cases, the body is punished and doesn't get the nutrients it needs to support normal cyclical functions. If this is sustained, biorhythms are severely disrupted, menstrual cycles disappear, and mental health issues may worsen or appear for the first time.

In exercise, undertraining and overtraining are signals that Scorpio's routine needs some help. When we're sedentary, we don't assist Scorpio in circulating and excreting waste through the skin and other emunctories. When we overtrain, we generate a huge amount of waste products for the body to sort through. Both extremes lead to the same place: the Scorpio body areas become overloaded and toxicity is retained. This is aggravated by Scorpio's tendency to get stuck in repetitive movement loops. This sign can latch on to high-intensity, low-intensity, or a single type of movement and not know when to let go. An extreme example being a runner who refuses to stop even though they're headed for a double knee replacement. All-or-nothing fitness approaches are severely damaging for Scorpio because they don't allow the body to go through normal energy fluctuations or repair cycles. They also block Scorpio from emotional maturation because they further encourage attachment to extreme states and experiences. Pushing through pain, slow workout recovery, and lingering injuries are signs that Scorpio's approach isn't working.

Other Planets in Scorpio
Mercury in Scorpio

Mercury in Scorpio's food mindset can be intense, but the upside is it usually has the drive to be intentional and organized with its nutrition. The microbiome's connection to cognition is highlighted, particularly in focus and problem-solving. This Mercury is prone to gut bugs, and consumption of garlic, ginger, turmeric, and other fresh herbs may be advisable for their antimicrobial action.

For this Mercury, a touch of perfectionism and paranoia can affect both the movement and food relationship. Mercury in Scorpio is often determined to follow a program to the letter, even if it's to their detriment. It can be wary of change and fixated on an approach even if it's no longer supportive. In some cases, the bowels or bladder can be hyperresponsive to movement.

Venus in Scorpio

The gut-hormone relationship is primary for Venus in Scorpio. It may be prone to estrogen-related imbalances, complicated by a susceptibility to candidiasis and other fungal infections. Candida thrives on starch and sugar. If experiencing these things, Venus in Scorpio may find a moderately low carbohydrate menu focusing on vegetables, protein, and fermented food to assist healing.

This Venus values intense emotional experiences and usually likes workouts to have a dramatic flair. This is great unless identity and self-worth become confused with extremes. The pelvic floor can sometimes be weak and need rehabilitation.

Mars in Scorpio

Fast-metabolizing Mars in Scorpio may have increased caloric and protein requirements. This placement may experience irritable bowel syndrome (IBS), inflammatory bowel disease (IBD), hemorrhoids, and other inflammatory conditions in the colon, bladder, or genitals. Optimizing fiber intake and identifying your personal inflammatory triggers, whether they be food-related, environmental, work-related, or emotional, may be necessary for healing.

This Mars is often competitive and goal- and task-oriented, and it tends to enjoy fitness programs that incorporate these elements. But it easily overdoes it, making it prone to injury and difficulty ridding itself of toxins, which may result in acne, body odor, headaches, changes in libido, and irritability.

Jupiter in Scorpio

Jupiter in Scorpio can accumulate dampness in the lower abdomen, making it prone to bacterial and fungal overgrowths in the GI. In some cases, other Scorpio body areas may see growths, such as uterine fibroids, ovarian cysts, or prostate enlargement. Like Venus in Scorpio, eating for a healthy gut-hormone relationship and temporarily adjusting carbohydrate consumption may be necessary during times of imbalance.

Regular doses of high-intensity movement that promote a healthy sweat can help keep this Jupiter's Water in bounds. Movement can be alchemical and often extends beyond the body into the realms of spiritual and personal development.

Saturn in Scorpio

Saturn in Scorpio may experience both functional issues and physical or emotional blockages in the GI, reproductive system, or pelvis generally. The relationship to fiber should be investigated, and if food sensitivities are present, be curious about mental-emotional and environmental contributors. This Saturn is long-suffering and may not reach out for professional help until a condition has progressed significantly.

Exercise is usually extremely helpful for this Saturn's mental health. Stress and pressure build up internally and, without an outlet, tend to crystallize and get shunted to other body systems. But this Saturn can push itself beyond its physical means and needs to take a balanced approach to movement. There can be structural issues in the pelvis, lower spine, and sacrum that require both decongesting the area and strengthening the surrounding muscles.

Uranus in Scorpio

Uranus may create disruption in any part of the Scorpio body, such as alternating constipation and diarrhea, bladder irritation or urinary incontinence, and sex hormone abnormalities. Supplemental soluble fiber is often a helpful Scorpio bowel and hormone stabilizer. The thyroid may have a role in any hormonal or digestive issues, as Uranus can irritate Taurus from across the zodiac.

This Uranus can be quite athletic and powerful, but it is prone to injury in the groin, sacrum, or coccyx.

Neptune in Scorpio

Neptune in Scorpio can create a general lack of tone in the organs of the lower abdomen, making it more prone to infection, toxicity, and deficiency. There may be excessive menstrual bleeding and cramps, prolapse, or hemorrhoids. Excess sugar and starch may aggravate this Neptune if it's experiencing candida overgrowth, vaginal yeast infections, and bladder or urinary tract infections.

Scorpio Nourishment Checklist	Scorpio Movement Checklist
Gesture: Transformation	**Gesture:** Power
+ Know your fibers	+ Intense but controlled
+ Pre- and probiotic foods	+ Stoke metabolism
+ Prioritize protein	+ Support healthy catharsis
+ Remember the gut-hormone relationship	+ Support sacrum, groin, and pelvis
+ Support detox organs	

PISCES

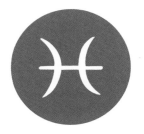

Pisces Anatomy

Pisces is most frequently compared to the ocean. Like the other Water signs, it primarily rules body fluids, where they gather, and how well they flow. Just as the ocean seems endless from the shore, the watery systems Pisces governs span vast distances in the body. What separates Pisces from the other Water signs is that it moves through the world in a mutable way. This means that it's not only endless Water but changing and traveling Water.

Mode	Ruling Planets
Mutable	**Jupiter** (traditional) **Neptune** (modern)

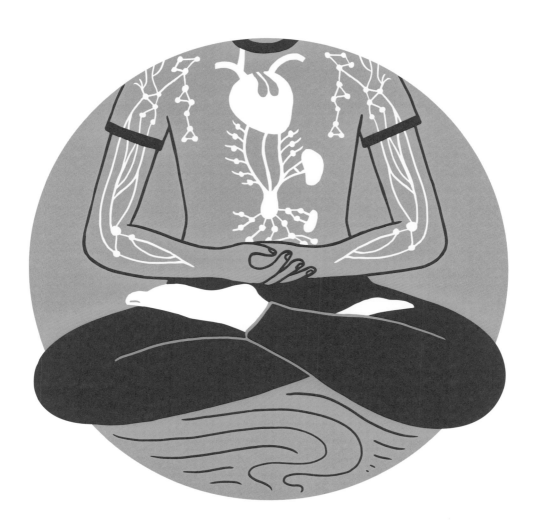

+ Feet

+ Lymphatic system (including lymph, vessels, ducts, and nodes)

+ Immune system (including all immune tissue found in the gut such as GALT, MALT, lacteals, and the appendix)

+ Small intestine

+ Blood (white blood cells, clotting ability, cholesterol content)

+ Energetic, emotional, and spiritual bodies

Pisces Nutrition

Gesture: Freedom

Pisces is a beautifully open sign. And while you never want to inhibit its freedom, you do want Pisces's Water to flow optimally. When Pisces's Water spreads too far without any sort of compassionate container, you may experience a breakdown of the body's integrity (see the imbalance list on page 109). This makes the body, mind, and spirit vulnerable to outside invasion and influence. Pisces nutrition is a dance between finding food joy and food freedom and keeping the body feeling maintained and protected. Let's take the ocean for example. It's vast and free but still has a container created by land. But the water doesn't stop exactly at the shore. It splashes up the coast and the tides reach up and down the beach. The water only goes so far, but its container is adaptable. It's possible for Pisces nutrition to be the same. You can create a health-supporting nutritional container for yourself without surrendering your freedom to hard noes and stiff limits.

Enforcing a bunch of food rules for Pisces typically doesn't go over too well. Sure, Pisces can follow a strict diet if it wants to. After all, it's partnered with Virgo. As much as Pisces may be inclined to throw all nutrition advice out the window, it's just as likely to overindulge in the militant food approach embraced by imbalanced Virgo energy. But I often witness Pisces people uncomfortably straddling both camps. When a diet ends, a stressful event occurs, or something slightly off-menu passes their lips, things tend to flood out of control quickly. And sadly, Pisces always blames itself instead of blaming the rigid and flawed dieting structure. A healthy food relationship often begins with Pisces knowing it's allowed to have what it wants. It needs to know it has the permission and freedom to choose its food, and that it can trust itself with that freedom. When this Jupiter-ruled sign is slapped with rigidity, its knee-jerk reaction will always be to expand, overextend, or push the limits even further. In a food context, this might mean eating or drinking to discomfort or not respecting your body with your food choices.

The tricky part is—like its partner sign, Virgo—Pisces often reports suffering from food allergies, intolerances, and sensitivities. Heightened sensitivity is one of the many ways Pisces may experience openness. This sensitivity might extend beyond food to how food is preserved, packaged, grown, raised, prepared, or spoken about. The subtle information carried in food and the subtle messages shared about food are not so subtle for Pisces. It's pretty common for Pisces to be on a self- or provider-prescribed elimination diet (where suspected trigger foods are removed) when I see them for the first time. Sure, this *might* be the right step for someone. But the issue is that, on a cellular and subconscious level, Pisces DNA often registers this practice as a loss in freedom and therefore an assault on its natural essence. What's missing from many elimination diets is healing the root cause. Often, a food is eliminated and that's that. Instead of promoting healing, this tends to promote food phobia. But barring a severe food allergy, a single food is not the root cause of a food sensitivity. For Pisces to get on board, it needs to be reminded of the big picture. If eliminating a food is appropriate, the elimination's purpose is to clarify and make space. Removing the food quiets the reactivity so that you can actually see what's underneath the reaction, and it gives the body room to heal. After that occurs, ideally the food is reintroduced and enjoyed again.

If you have a condition that requires medical nutrition therapy, it's still important to cultivate a feeling of freedom. I've had to reframe the concept of freedom quite a bit in my own life as I've navigated different health challenges. For me, freedom also means willingly choosing some foods over others to increase my quality of life, create a more pleasant physical experience, and minimize pain and discomfort. Willingness is the secret ingredient, as is emphasizing that I always have the freedom to choose differently if I want to. If that definition of freedom doesn't resonate with you, I encourage you to play with this concept until you find something that does.

Pisces and Mold

Pisces may discover it's highly sensitive to micro amounts of mold and mycotoxins, thanks to its damp nature and modern ruler Neptune. Some amount of mold is typically found on nuts, seeds, and grains. Pick through, rinse, or soak nuts, seeds, and grains and then dry nuts at a low temperature in the oven or a dehydrator. Bulk bins are often prone to storage mold growth. For very prone foods such as cashews, peanuts, wheat, oats, and corn, it may be best to find a reputable source that third-party tests for mycotoxins. Pisces often likes a little coffee to keep it going, but coffee beans are also prone to mycotoxins. If you drink a lot of coffee and are highly sensitive, it may be worth splurging on beans that have been tested. If you opt for decaf, try water processed, as the chemicals used in caffeine extraction often leave Pisces feeling fuzzy.

Pisces's openness can sometimes express as increased vulnerability to catching a cold or other infection. Consciously eating to support the immune system may be a wise choice. Stock up on vegetables and fruits high in vitamin C; incorporate foods with anti-inflammatory or immune-modulating effects, such as garlic, ginger, and mushrooms; and add more selenium- and zinc-containing foods to your plate. Brazil nuts are a wonderful source of selenium, while legumes, seeds (especially hemp and pumpkin), shellfish, and red meat all have a hefty amount of zinc. Don't forget the immune system's massive presence in the gut (ruled by Pisces). Regularly supplement with foods that support the gut lining and microbiome, such as bone broth and fermented vegetables.

Eating for blood, mood, and sleep is another Pisces nutritional foundation. From a Chinese Medicine perspective, these three things are deeply intertwined. The concept of blood extends well beyond the stuff circulating in our vessels. It nourishes the physical body, but it's also an anchoring fluid for the spirit. If blood is weak, the spirit gets restless, leading to mental-emotional discomfort and sleep disturbances. Enriching the blood is immensely important considering that many Pisces-dominant people report heightened sensitivity, fatigue, depression, pathological empathy, or simply feeling out of body. Sometimes this is complicated by Pisces's tendency to follow a vegetarian or vegan diet, which when not carefully planned, may be too low in blood-supporting nutrients. I've talked to many vegetarian Pisceans who have reluctantly reintroduced animal protein into their diet to heal their body and give themselves a measure of grounding, but they continue to have an aversion to red meat and rely on poultry and fish. Regardless of the dietary path you choose, Pisces thrives on a variety of plant foods rich in iron, vitamin B_{12}, and folate, particularly dark leafy greens, seaweeds, algae, and sprouts. Cook in cast-iron pots to add more iron to your diet, and if you eat animal protein, incorporate regular red meat, organ meats, chicken, eggs, and gelatin to nourish the blood.

Protecting Sleep

Pisces often needs more sleep than the other signs. It's completely normal and healthy for Pisces to need ten or more hours of sleep per night. If you struggle with insomnia, experiment with your evening foods and food timing. Try making your last meal easily digestible and avoid going to bed feeling overfull. On the other hand, if you're eating your last meal many hours before bedtime, a drop in blood sugar may be keeping you awake. Blackout curtains, blue-light blocking glasses, sleep masks, and noise-canceling headphones are Pisces's best friends.

Pisces Movement

Gesture: Fluidity

As vast as the ocean, the ways this sign expresses itself in movement are almost innumerable. Pisces is so mutable and easily immersed that it often picks up movement easily, almost like osmosis. Of course, we see Pisces in water sports such as swimming or surfing, but this sign takes the attributes of Water to any movement it touches. Pisces movers are often skilled in, or at least interested in, several different sports or events and how they combine— one example, being a triathlete. They also tend to be attracted to fusions of fitness and spirituality or mindfulness as we see in yogic traditions, tai chi, and qi gong. Contortion and feats of flexibility and balance are also very Piscean and may show up in acrobatics, gymnastics, or slacklining. And we can't forget the involvement of the feet in soccer, tap dancing, ballet, and barefoot sports of all kinds. Pisces has its feet in a lot of different things.

Many Pisces-dominant people prefer yoga, dance, or bodyweight movement, but because Pisces tends to be overly open emotionally and physically, it's also important for this sign to intentionally create fortitude. Astrological exercise expands beyond the body, and you can use it to bolster signs' weaknesses. You want to keep Pisces graceful and flexible, but make sure it's not porous or vulnerable to outside influences. This means regularly incorporating strength or corrective work into the routine and ensuring that the often hypermobile Pisces body is keeping proper positions while moving.

Head to clairegallagher.co/bodyastro for video examples of Pisces movements.

Pisces Strength and Conditioning

Although difficult in its own way, Pisces strength and conditioning typically isn't going to leave you on the floor heaving for breath. Instead, the focus is to embody Water, meaning that rather than aiming for heaviness or speed, training is more skill-based and uses elements of rotation, balance, flexibility, and pivoting elegantly through many positions, such as from lying to kneeling, kneeling to standing, and back again. Although quickness is sometimes needed as a tool to wake up Pisces, for the majority of the time, Pisces routines are unhurried and timeless, allowing it to focus more on form and sensation.

In the gym, Pisces's niche is fluid strength. Pisces strength work isn't clunky or disjointed; it's a dance too, just involving weight. My favorite way to develop fluid strength is through a combination of kettlebell and bodyweight flows. The ballistic motion of a kettlebell requires extreme power, balance, and control, but a skilled practitioner can make maneuvering the heaviest bells look smooth and effortless. A kettlebell flow is created by stringing multiple movements into a fluid dance. Similarly, floor flows are often sequences of postures strung together. They may be yogic or animal-inspired, and they typically keep your body very close to the ground, often requiring a lot of hip flexibility and upper body strength.

Foot position is another pillar of Pisces training. For injury prevention and movement longevity, focus on form from the ground up. When Pisces movers have their foot position right, the upstream structures tend to align. Once you have the basics down, experiment with alternative and asymmetrical foot positioning, such as staggered stances and elevating the toes or heels. If safe and permissible, do your workout barefoot to allow for deeper sensory connection with the feet and for an added balance challenge.

Pisces Running

Because they're both mutable and ruled by expansive Jupiter, Pisces and Sagittarius share a similar interest in running that's freeing and exploratory. Where they differ is that Pisces is a Water sign, which brings a cooler nature to its approach. I've known a handful of Pisces marathoners. Their attraction to the sport rarely lies in speed or winning and more often lies in the hypnotic, meandering length of the race and training schedule. Running tends to act as a peaceful and transcendent escape for this sign. Another large factor in Pisces running is, of course, the feet. This has a wide range of manifestations and may show up as an interest in barefoot running, a love of intricate footwork, structural foot issues requiring orthotics, or just a huge collection of shoes. Running near water or just taking long walks is great for Pisces too. Regardless of this sign's preferred type of exercise, walking supports the increased global blood and lymph flow that it often needs.

Pisces Yoga

Although all yoga practices focus on grounding through the feet, a Pisces practice has an extra measure of foot awareness. Prioritize spreading the toes and placing equal pressure in all corners of the feet, and if you can, keep your feet warm. Lymph and blood flow are especially important for this sign. A well-rounded Pisces routine will incorporate plenty of opportunities to get the feet above the head. Toe stands and balancing postures of all kinds carry a natural Pisces imprint, as do trancelike flows that allow you to get lost in the motion. Because of the increased flexibility, balance, and creative use of the feet, AcroYoga is another Pisces favorite.

Other Pisces Sports and Classes

- ✦ Ballet or pointe
- ✦ Circus arts
- ✦ Deepwater running
- ✦ Diving
- ✦ Fly-fishing

- ✦ Kickball
- ✦ Soccer
- ✦ Step dance
- ✦ Surfing

- ✦ Synchronized swimming
- ✦ Tap dance
- ✦ Triathlon
- ✦ Waterskiing

Pisces Conditions

Jupiter and Neptune are responsible for Pisces's expansive and endless nature. Jupiter is buoyant and growth-oriented, and Neptune seeks to transcend definition, boundary, and structure. These qualities are at the root of Pisces's greatest gifts and deepest struggles. The most common Pisces imbalances begin when physical or spiritual resources expand, seep, or leak beyond the safe container of the body. Over time, this breaks down the integrity of the body and we can feel overstretched, weakened, and vulnerable. This porousness opens the body to both physical and spiritual invasion. Like pulling from a poisoned well, resources become contaminated and circulate their effects throughout the body. Pisces conditions may manifest as:

Autoimmune disease

Bloating, diarrhea, and food reactions that express in systems outside of the gastrointestinal tract or in the emotional body

Blood-borne, vector-borne, and water-borne illnesses (E. coli, giardia, hepatitis, Lyme disease,

salmonella)

Chronic fatigue syndrome related to a prior viral infection such as Epstein-Barr virus, psychic attack, or spiritual crisis

Corns, bunions, athlete's foot, swelling, pain, injury, or structural abnormality in the feet

Depression

Hypermobility and Ehlers-Danlos syndrome

Immune system deficiency and catching cold frequently

Lymphedema and stagnation, water retention

Mysterious, often misdiagnosed illnesses and psychosomatic conditions

Poor circulation, anemias, clotting disorders, menorrhagia, high cholesterol, high blood sugar, atherosclerosis

Sleep disturbances (insomnia, night terrors, narcolepsy, sleepwalking, somnolence, vivid dreams)

Undulating beneath most Pisces food and movement imbalances is a lack of anchoring and trust in the body. Pisces has often dealt with so much sensitivity, fatigue, confusion, or illness that they feel betrayed by the body and may feel safer living outside of it. In a daily fitness and nutrition scenario, this might show up as a lack of clarity in how to exercise or what to eat or a feeling of overwhelm with the many different choices. A primary part of healing the Pisces food and movement relationship is repairing self-trust and clearing the line of communication with the body. If there's already a clear exchange with the body, the task is usually to follow the inner wisdom received instead of disregarding it. Pisces is often up for trying anything and everything, but if it doesn't have that anchoring and clarity within itself, it's easily influenced by external opinions. It will often get swept away by a very extreme approach, waking up a few months later totally drained, or take a directionless approach that's too diluted to deliver the benefits it's seeking.

Not being fully anchored in the body may also manifest as not honoring your own limits. Jupiter-ruled Pisces can easily overdo anything, and may be overly optimistic about its body's capacity, finding itself exhausted for the next week because it did too much. On the other hand, Pisces may not know when it's safe to push and work a little bit harder. To make things even more confusing, Pisces typically finds itself fluctuating between this chronic overdoing and underdoing.

Being in a Pisces body can sometimes feel very inconsistent and unpredictable. But all astrological bodies have unique energetic patterns and Pisces is no different. Seeing, validating, and living within your own energetic flow are immensely important for every sign. But this is often exceptionally challenging for Pisces (and most Water bodies, for that matter) because our boxy world doesn't recognize the circular wisdom of this sign. It's normal for Pisces to have large energetic fluctuations, just like the ocean's tides. These fluctuations are part of Pisces's structure, it's just that the structure is a fluid one.

When Pisces people tell me they have no discipline or drive and that if left to their own devices they'd never exercise or eat healthfully, this is usually a cultural judgment that they've internalized. If Pisces tries to make their food and movement approach fit into a rigid box, it typically won't work long term because it's inherently self-rejecting. When the body's natural flow is rejected, this is when Pisces may find itself self-sabotaging its health efforts or engaging in escapist behavior. Healing this involves fully accepting how its body functions, learning that living in its own flow isn't dangerous or less than, and designing a food and movement approach that leaves plenty of space to unfold differently day to day without judgment.

Other Planets in Pisces
Mercury in Pisces

Mercury in Pisces is more prone to depression, overwhelm, foggy brain, nervousness, and abnormal sleep patterns than others. Eating for cognitive, mood, and sleep health is a priority. Fatty acids may be important for keeping this Mercury afloat, and targeted amino acid supplementation could be helpful.

The desire or ability to exercise may be highly variable. Use flexible parameters within workouts, such as set, rep, rest, and weight ranges. Ranges allow you to maintain an overarching program direction, but they also offer the flexibility to shift small variables in a workout to match your current energetic state. Sometimes this Mercury is hypermobile and needs to focus on carefully maintaining position integrity during exercise.

Venus in Pisces

The sugar relationship may be complicated for tenderhearted Venus in Pisces and could range from simply having a sweet tooth to dealing with fructose sensitivity or general carb malabsorption. There may be an excess amount of Water in the body, which from an elemental medicine perspective could contribute to hormonal imbalances. Eating plenty of healthy fats for hormonal health is often necessary.

This Venus is a very intuitive mover and naturally drawn to yoga or dance. It often desires exercise to double as a spiritual or emotional expression.

But because this is such a soft and energetically porous placement, it's also important that some measure of fortitude be brought into the routine via traditional strength training or another grounding form of exercise.

Mars in Pisces

Mars in Pisces's immune system is often hyperreactive and may have what feels like disproportionate reactions to small stimuli or even autoimmune reactions. Responses are histamine heavy and feel like a large rush of heat, often leading to insomnia and mental anguish. This Mars often needs help moving toxicity out of the body and may need to explore food allergens.

This Mars easily pushes past its own movement limits. Even if it doesn't feel like too much at the time, it's common for this placement to go a little too hard and suffer a negative immune or hormonal response to intense exercise. Programs should have built-in gradations and fluctuations to keep you moving without having to endure uncomfortable setbacks.

Jupiter in Pisces

Unlike the deficient picture of many other planets in Pisces, Jupiter in Pisces is often overly abundant. High blood sugar, high cholesterol, or water retention are possible complaints. Liver function may be sluggish, and eating liver-loving foods and optimizing liver function are important in helping this Jupiter feel free and unburdened.

Because this Jupiter tends to hold on to so much water, some amount of regular sweating is encouraged. When excess water builds up in this system, any existing sugar, blood, or liver imbalances could be exaggerated.

Saturn in Pisces

Saturn in Pisces may suffer with depression, anemia, menstrual irregularities, poor blood or lymph circulation, deficient immune response, or sluggish function of both the liver and gut. It needs a very warming, nutrient-dense diet that's extremely easy to digest. Prioritize foods rich in iron, vitamin B_{12}, folate, and protein that support mood and blood.

It's very important that this Saturn learns to love and accept its waxing and waning bodily experience. If the exercise routine doesn't account for normal body fluctuations, it's possible to feel completely exhausted by movement. Excessive sweating, such as what's experienced in hot yoga, should be handled with care. This Saturn needs to be built up with exercise, instead of depleted. This may mean less cardio, less sweating, and more strengthening and building of the body's structure.

Uranus in Pisces

Uranus in Pisces may experience large fluctuations in the body waters, which not only includes fluids but also hormones and emotions. Poor carbohydrate metabolism and blood sugar dysregulation may be present. Somewhat like Mercury in Pisces, this Uranus often does well with an overarching training direction but with plenty of room for variation and intuitive movement. Be sure to investigate foot positioning and structure if any pain is present during exercise.

Neptune in Pisces

Neptune in Pisces may experience mysterious illnesses, lingering fatigue, multiple allergies, and meandering symptoms of all kinds. Healing often requires immune strengthening, gut repair, and fortifying the energetic and spiritual bodies. Vigorous exercise may feel unnatural for this placement but may be a helpful stimulant. Don't skimp on athletic footwear—make sure you have something supportive.

Pisces Nourishment Checklist	Pisces Movement Checklist
Gesture: Freedom	**Gesture:** Fluidity
✦ Eat for immunity	✦ Foot positioning and awareness
✦ Explore the root cause	✦ Fluid strength
✦ Food permission and allowance	✦ Rotating, balancing, and pivoting
✦ Honor sensitivity	✦ Spiritual movement fusions
✦ Iron-rich foods	✦ Support lymph and blood flow
✦ Support sleep	✦ Unhurried and hypnotic

THE
PLANETS

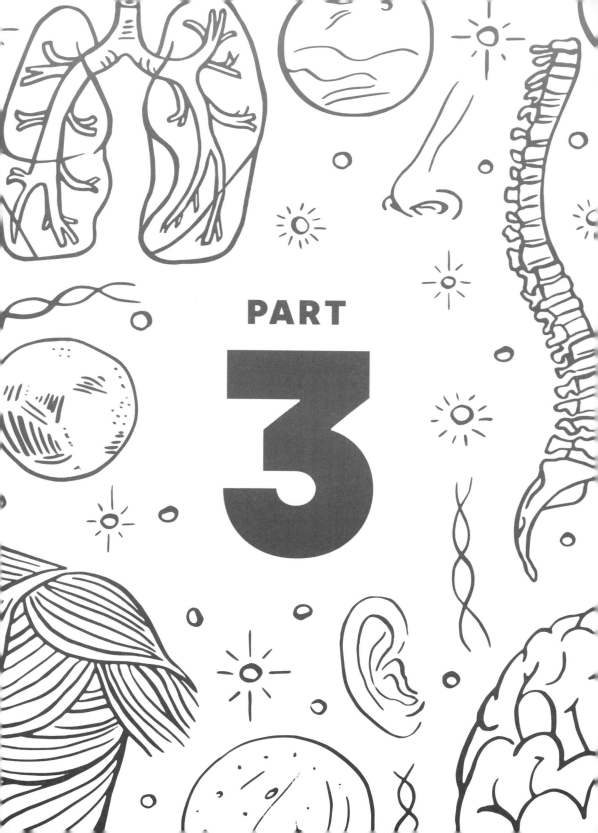

PART

3

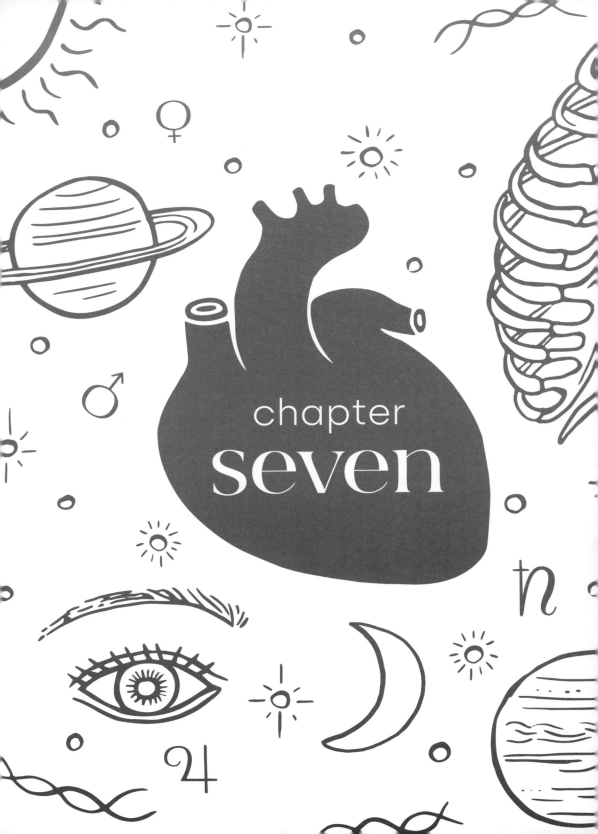

chapter
seven

USING THE PLANETS TO HEAL

Planet refresher: They move through the zodiac signs and create change. They're the action in astrology. Saturn constricts. Mercury connects. Venus relaxes. Your birth chart is a snapshot of where the planets were when you were born. The signs tell us where and how these actions are taking place in the body.

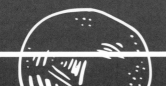

Your birth chart describes your astro-genetics, but to understand how your body and life change over time, you must look to today's sky. After you were born, the planets kept moving, creating new celestial weather patterns and energetic systems. This motion and how it interacts with your birth chart are what astrologers call transits. I bet you've heard of one specific transit before. The famous Saturn return, when Saturn in the real-time sky returns to where it was when you were born, is a transit. Saturn is slow. Your first Saturn return happens when you're about twenty-nine years old and lasts for around two years. Your second Saturn return happens around fifty-eight and, for some, again twenty-nine years later. These periods of life are often very defining. During the first Saturn return, many people are beginning careers, going to school, starting families or businesses, or establishing their life paths in other ways. It's like a celestial coming of age. The second Saturn return revisits these themes slightly differently. Maybe you're changing careers, getting ready to retire, watching your kids have kids, or experiencing another transition. These transits are thresholds. From a health perspective, Saturn transits can be quite stressful and physically demanding, and we often need extra nutrients to stay the course. But a Saturn return is just one of many transits. It just happens to be the most well known—other than Mercury retrograde, of course.

In the following pages, we're going to take a deep dive into each planet's physical role and needs, or what each planet may require to stay healthy and feeling like itself. The information in each planet's section is intended to help you come back to baseline, or even completely bust free when you feel buried or lost in a transit.

Transit Care 101

Planetary transits commonly coincide with life seasons that require different nutrition and self-care from our norm. For example, we need unique nourishment in childhood versus our teens, in winter versus summer, and in pregnancy versus menopause. It's the same with transits. Transits define new physical needs. Saturn transits need different nutrition from Jupiter transits, and Venus transits need different movement from Mars transits. Transits also define new emotional needs. Within food and movement, this might mean kindly adjusting our self-talk and expectations. Ultimately, transits give us a new, more compassionate lens with which to look at our life.

We're constantly undergoing planetary transits. Some transits last years and some last days. They can define entire chapters of life or simply the essence of a single week. As the planets move through the sky, our bodies are presented with new information to filter and assimilate. Sometimes we integrate transits easily and our lives may reflect this back to us with good health, new opportunities, and general well-being. But sometimes planetary energy is just tough to integrate and we might experience pain, grief, illness, or other types of suffering.

The great news is that over time, taking care of your natal chart transforms you into a planetary processing machine. Having the right tools and habits in place to keep your astrological body generally balanced makes you more resilient and likely to process changing cosmic energy with efficiency and ease. But, inevitably, larger, slower, and more powerful transits happen. This is when you may need to reach beyond the birth chart and work with a particular planet.

Here's the thing—planetary energy is going to express no matter what, but I believe we have a say in how. For example, let's say we've pinpointed Mars as the planet coinciding with a bout of severe inflammation we're having. Mars's energy is expressing through our body. Mars will never stop expressing, and we don't want it to. After all, Mars is what also gives us drive and passion. But in this case, we'd love for Mars to express in a more constructive way. To get its attention and redirect its power, we can use a Mars-flavored food and movement approach or that of its balancing planet (more on that in a bit).

When we fill our lives with food, movement, and activities that correspond with a planet's natural personality and agenda, we're essentially flagging it down and enticing it to get on our side and work with us. When we stop viewing ourselves as subject to astrological whims and instead direct difficult planetary energy in new ways, the planet now has other ways to manifest beyond symptoms and challenging circumstances. Now we get to use this planet's power to heal and the planet still gets to express its natural energy. It's a win-win.

The Sovereign Astrology Mindset

Before we go on, I want to be very clear—I don't believe planets create disease or misfortune. This way of thinking creates a lot of unhelpful astrological fear. When we label certain planets or transits as "good" or "bad," we severely limit the many ways they could unfold. I like to keep my options open, and I prefer to relate to planetary transits as opportunities. You are in charge of how you respond to everything, and that includes transits.

When first diving into physical astrology, it's easy to get stuck in a pattern of always looking for what's wrong. Learn from my mistakes—planetary transits also inform us about current opportunities for more joy and expansion.

Transits aren't synonymous with difficulty. It's equally likely for a transit to coincide with growth opportunities, and it's our choice whether we reach out for them and participate.

Picking a Planet

Don't worry, you don't have to be an astrologer to know which planet to start with. Knowing how to identify transits can make this practice extremely powerful, but until you get there, you can just as easily rely on all the body wisdom and intuition you already have. There are three ways to explore the planets: using intuition, body clues, or astrology to identify transits.

If you aren't sure what transits you're undergoing, but you know that something feels off, I highly encourage you to **use your intuition** to choose a planet. Intuition speaks to each of us in unique ways. Some hear it, some see it, some write it, some speak it, some feel it, and some of us "just know." When using intuition to choose a planet, allow it to come forward in the normal way you'd relate to your intuitive voice. Nothing special required. I also encourage you to pay attention to any planets that you're simply attracted to or most interested in. These are clues. Investigate them.

Your body is extremely wise and constantly showering you with information. New or returning symptoms that you thought you resolved are always clues. If you notice your normal patterns shifting or new things popping up in your body, you can bet a planetary cycle is linked to it. To use **body clues**, read through the planets until you identify something that resembles your current symptom pattern and life experience, or use the "Symptoms" appendix in the back of the book for direction.

With a bit more astrological know-how, you can pick your planet with precision by **identifying the transits** you're currently experiencing. There are so many amazing apps and programs these days that will list your transits for you—no need to even spend time deciphering your chart (see the resources section for a few suggestions). But we're often undergoing so many transits at once that even a simple list can be overwhelming. Here are a few transit basics to help guide your choice.

Not all transits are major. Give priority to any transits affecting the major pieces of your astro-genetics. Remember from chapter 1, the absolute essentials are your Sun, Moon, and rising sign.

Some planets move fast. The Sun, Moon, Mercury, Venus, and Mars are speedy and may change signs multiple times per month. These transits may last only a day or two and usually don't require anything massive. But if one of these planets changes direction (stations retrograde or stations direct), or if there's an eclipse on an important part of your chart, you may want to get to know that planet better.

Some planets move slow. Jupiter, Saturn, Uranus, Neptune, and Pluto take their time moving around the zodiac. When one of these planets transits a piece of your birth chart, you'll feel it for a few months or up to a few years and you may experience significant changes. Prioritize these.

Care for the planet being transited first. A transit involves two players: the transiting planet in the real-time sky and your natal planet being transited. For example, maybe transiting Saturn is activating your natal Moon. Which one do you pay attention to? Usually the natal planet is the one that needs strengthening and attention (in this case, the Moon). But it's not a bad idea to look at both planets' sections and see which one feels more accurate or to take a combo approach.

Some transits are harder than others. The geometrical relationships or angles between the planets are called "aspects." The type of aspect between a transiting planet and your natal planet shows how their different energies might work together. Just like human relationships, some planetary relationships are smoother than others. Prioritizing transits that involve aspects such as a conjunction, opposition, square, or inconjunct is important because these are the ones that usually require physical attention. Keep in mind, planets send their vibes in all different directions and a transiting planet does *not* have to be in the same zodiac sign as a natal planet to be affecting it.

Using Planetary Energy Like a Pro

Timing

Though transits last a specific length of time, they don't feel the same that entire time. Transits increase and decrease in strength. To avoid overwhelm, I suggest saving planetary adjustments to your self-care for when a transit is strongest. The closer a transiting planet is to your natal planet, the more noticeable it is.

How do you know when a transit is at its strongest? You can rely on life clues, but you can also use astro-math. If you look at your birth chart, you'll see little numbers next to your natal planets. These are their exact degree and minute locations, or zodiac addresses. Let's pretend your natal Moon lives at the 28th degree of Sagittarius. If transiting Mars is only at the 5th degree of Sagittarius, it's 23 degrees away from your Moon and probably too far off to be felt. But when it gets to around the 23rd degree of Sagittarius, and especially the 28th degree, you're going to feel it. Astrological opinions differ greatly, but for simplicity, I find that most people feel transits within 5 degrees of a natal planet on either side (sometimes a little less on the back end).

Transit Pulsing

For very long transits, I suggest pulsing your approach, meaning to go in and out of using the suggestions in its corresponding section(s). Focus on these suggestions when a transit is at its peak, but for the rest of the time, revisit them only when you feel it's necessary or when a longer transit is activated by shorter transits. For example, a Pluto transit may last three years, but this doesn't mean you should do Pluto therapeutics that entire time. Over that three-year period, the transit will wax and wane in intensity and get activated by smaller astrological events happening nearby, such as Full Moons, eclipses, or faster planets like Mars and Mercury zooming by. These moments are when you might want to pulse your approach and revisit the Pluto suggestions for a few days. If that's too much astrology for you, fall back on using your body clues and intuition to determine when the transit intensity is high. Or simply pulse at regular intervals for maintenance, such as every three months, until the transit is over, or whatever feels right to you.

Planetary Balancing

When planets act on the body, we usually experience the symptoms as too much (excess) or too little (deficiency). To make planetary information easier to use, I've categorized symptoms as excess or deficient, but in reality, the lines aren't so clear. Excess and deficiency are less of a line and more of a dynamic circle. When a planet creates excess for too long, we eventually become fatigued and show signs of deficiency. And when a planet creates deficiency for too long, things can stagnate, build up, and eventually express as excess. Mixed pictures are possible. It's likely you'll identify yourself on both sides, especially during a long transit.

If a planet is deficient, we usually need more of it. For example, if Mars is weak, we'd use Mars tools to strengthen it. But if Mars is too strong, adding more Mars would make the problem worse. Instead, we need to balance it with opposing planetary forces. Within each planet's section, I've given you its balancing planets and explained which one is most appropriate to use when, but you can also use the summarized table on page 223.

How Long Do Transits Last?

The length of a transit depends on how fast a planet is moving and if a retrograde is in its future. If a planet stations (pauses before changing direction) retrograde or direct near one of your natal planets, the transit length increases significantly. But transit length is also determined by your personal sensitivity to planetary energy, as well as how much influence you choose to give the planets in degrees (see the discussion on timing). This table reflects my personal felt experience with transits and how I've seen them unfold in professional practice. Experiences differ, so use it as a ballpark idea.

APPROXIMATE TRANSIT LENGTH

Planet	Length
Sun	1–3 days
Moon	1–2 days
Mercury	2–7 days
Venus	1–2 weeks
Mars	2 weeks–1 month
Jupiter	2–3 months
Saturn	1.5–3 years
Uranus	2 years
Neptune	3 years
Pluto	3 years

Planetary Balancing

Planet	Balance/Reduce with
Sun	Not recommended
Moon	Saturn, Mars
Mercury	Jupiter, Venus, Saturn, Neptune
Venus	Mars, Mercury, Saturn, Uranus
Mars	Venus, Moon, Saturn, Neptune
Jupiter	Mercury, Saturn
Saturn	Sun, Mercury, Moon, Venus, Jupiter, Uranus, Neptune
Uranus	Venus, Saturn
Neptune	Mercury, Mars, Saturn
Pluto	Sun

I give much more information about Mercury, Venus, and Mars excess and deficiency because, beyond the Sun and Moon, they're the easiest to feel and understand, and you may cycle through these experiences several times throughout the astrological year. I didn't categorize Uranus, Neptune, and Pluto's conditions because they're too complex for this simplified model. They're strong forces that almost always act in excess. Their suggestions are designed to help you process and direct these forces in the most benefi-cial ways.

How to Use the Planetary Food Lists

Each planet's section also includes a food list. Most of these are very old astrological food associations from around the seventeenth century, but I've taken some creative liberty and added a few of my own. Although these traditional associations between planets, signs, and foods can be fascinating, we can run into a few snags when we get stuck on them. You may see the same food on multiple lists, but for different astrological reasons. For example, there are many opinions on which planet rules sweet potato, and none of them are wrong. We could say Venus because it's sweet and comforting. We could say the Moon because it grows in the damp earth. But we could also say Saturn for the same reason. Maybe the sweet potato's ruler really is Venus because it's carbohydrate heavy. Or perhaps it's the Sun because it's orange and high in vitamin A. Does this astrological rabbit trail help anyone? Probably not.

If I were to take these ancient associations very literally, I could make a leap like: Mars is deficient in this chart, so I only want you to eat Mars-ruled alliums and spices for a month. Or there's a Pisces problem going on here, so please load up on fish, alcohol, and sugar. This would create major distress in your digestive system. These examples are exaggerative, but the point is, just because a food belongs to a sign does *not* mean it's therapeutic for someone of that sign to consume it. Or consider this more serious example: Virgo may rule wheat, but my most frequently gluten-intolerant clients are dominant in Virgo or its partner sign, Pisces.

I like to think of the chart as a map of both the mental-emotional and physical food relationships and how we can repair those relationships. *Sometimes* that means looking at foods traditionally associated with a particular planet, but it always means compassionately addressing any underlying and painful food talk and supporting the chart's unique physiology. In a real astro-nutrition context, I *rarely* pay attention to the minutia of which food belongs to which sign or planet. Instead, I focus on the therapeutic gestures, or imprints of the signs and planets, and how I can mimic those gestures most appropriately for the person in front of me. And I encourage you to adopt this same mindset when looking at the planetary food lists for yourself. For example, the nutritional gesture of Mars is to heat. We could achieve this with Mars-ruled coffee and hot peppers—and maybe create some stomach-aches and stressed adrenals along the way—or with a stew full of warming spices. Perhaps the stew ingredients aren't traditionally ruled by Mars, but the temperature, seasoning, and protein content of the dish still carries a therapeutic Mars gesture (and one that's much more medicinal).

Food Allergies, Sensitivities, and Intolerances

I've also included a section on potential allergens and trouble foods for each planet. These come from my own research and practice in astro-nutrition. But before we explore this, I want to be very clear about my food sensitivity philosophy. Unfortunately, I've noticed that it's become rather common practice to blame any mysterious digestive complaint or symptom on a food sensitivity or intolerance—usually without accurate testing or diagnosis. I've also noticed that "wellness" culture has co-opted the idea of food sensitivity and erroneously related it to weight gain or loss. But food sensitivity is a *symptom* of something deeper. Additionally, sometimes what we're "intolerant" to isn't a food at all, but the difficult thoughts, feelings, and judgments surrounding eating. Food reactions are very real, and I'm not claiming otherwise. But I don't believe eliminating food is the first step in nutritional care, and I often see it do more harm than good. There are *so* many other things to address before eliminating foods. And although I have included this information in my book, I hope it's the last thing you consider.

So, how do you know if one of the foods on a planetary food list is aggravating you? Your body's signals are the best place to start, but from an astrological perspective, we can look to a concept called "planetary condition." Think of "planetary condition" as a list of criteria telling us how "happy" or "unhappy" a planet is in a particular location. This is important because "unhappy" planets are more likely to correlate with health imbalances (in this case, food sensitivities). This is how a planet can both rule a food and be troubled by that same food. For example, a "happy" Venus may be able to drink all the milk in the world, while an "unhappy" Venus may be lactose intolerant. It depends on that planet's condition in *your* chart. A planet's condition hinges on all sorts of things. Is it retrograde? Is it aspected by Saturn or Mars? (It can get complicated!) But the best place to start is just knowing what zodiac sign a planet is in and if it likes being there or not.

Remember the concept of planetary rulers from chapter 1? Each planet rules a sign (or two) and gives them their qualities and characteristics. The sign that a planet rules is called its *domicile*—just think of this sign as the

Planet	Domicile/ Rulership	Exaltation	Detriment	Fall
Sun	Leo	Aries	Aquarius	Libra
Moon	Cancer	Taurus	Capricorn	Scorpio
Mercury	Gemini/Virgo	Virgo*	Sagittarius/Pisces	Pisces**
Venus	Taurus/Libra	Pisces	Aries/Scorpio	Virgo
Mars	Aries/Scorpio	Capricorn	Taurus/Libra	Cancer
Jupiter	Sagittarius/Pisces	Cancer	Gemini/Virgo	Capricorn
Saturn	Capricorn/ Aquarius	Libra	Cancer/Leo	Aries

* Some authors say Aquarius.

** Some authors say Leo.

planet's home. Planets love hanging out at home, or in the sign they rule. Planets also like hanging out in the homes of their friends, also known as the signs they're *exalted in*. Planets aren't as comfortable in their signs of *detriment* or *fall*, but don't let these terms scare you. It just means that these planets may need more care and attention. If one of your natal planets is in detriment or fall, you *might* want a peek at the allergen list.

Use the above chart to see if any of your natal planets are more comfortable or uncomfortable. By the way, if you don't find any matches, that's totally normal.

Pro tip: Planets in their home signs can sometimes get too comfortable and correspond with excess conditions. For example, Mercury in Gemini can be witty and smart, but may experience things such as mental agitation, overwhelm, and stress. Even though Mercury rules Gemini, the body doesn't always register it as a pleasant experience.

The outer planets were discovered many years after these principles were created, but their modern signs of rulership, or home signs, are Aquarius (Uranus), Pisces (Neptune), and Scorpio (Pluto).

One last tip: Take a look at the food lists corresponding with the sign of your natal Mars and Saturn. These planets are the most likely to create physical imbalances. For example, if you have natal Mars in Leo, check out the Sun list. Since Leo is ruled by the Sun, it's also associated with the Sun's foods. Or, if your natal Saturn is in Scorpio, take a look at the Mars list; Mars rules Scorpio. You may notice a few trouble foods on these lists, *especially* if Mars or Saturn is retrograde, in a house of health, or aspects your natal Sun, Moon, or ascendant degree. I told you this could go deep! As always, start with the most basic layer and work from there.

SUN
Brightening

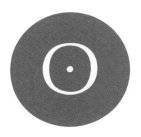

The Sun represents our vital force, that magic spark that keeps us alive. It's pure yang energy. The light of the Sun enlivens the body and awakens consciousness. It individuates us and gives us our sense of self and purpose.

Sun Basics

Rules: Leo

Element: Fire

Qualities: Hot, dry

Key Action: Animating, enlivening, tonifying, awakening

Body Functions: Heart function, consciousness, temperature regulation, sight, metabolism (with Mars and Saturn)

Solar Imbalances

Deficiency Not Vital Enough	Shared	Excess Distorted Vitality
Changes in eyesight Congenital disorders Dangerously low body temperature Depression, listlessness, lifelessness Loss of consciousness, fainting, confusion, coma Poor sense of self	Altered consciousness Heart disease Identity crisis Life force endangered Palpitations	Dangerously high body temperature Grandiose or narcissistic sense of self

Planetary Balancing

STRENGTHEN WITH	BALANCE WITH
More Sun Your Sun sign or the current Sun sign	In most cases, it's not recommended to reduce the Sun because it's your life force.

Solar Food and Movement

Solar food and movement brighten the mood, improve energy, and connect you back to your truest self. The best way to care for your natal Sun is to use the self-care information in your Sun sign's section. Although we can give the Sun a few of its own food and movement correlations, when your Sun needs a boost, it's more personal and practical to attend to the parts of the body that your natal Sun expresses through. Beyond the symptoms listed on page 229, if you experience any symptoms on your Sun sign's imbalance list, it's a clue that your Sun needs some strengthening. I also highly recommend strengthening your natal Sun if it's being transited by Saturn, Neptune, or Pluto.

On its own, the Sun has a natural correlation with cardiovascular exercise because it's the life-sustaining power of the heart. But instead of making your heart pump out of your chest (which is more Mars-like), Sun cardio is often moderate and supports mood and blood flow. This could be a nature walk, a leisurely run with your dog, playing with your kids, or having a kitchen dance party. If it gets you moving and lifts your spirits, it's good for your Sun. Extra cosmic points if you can do this movement in the sunshine. As the ruler of consciousness, the Sun is also nourished by movement and spirituality fusions.

As the Sun rotates around your birth chart each year, it also highlights and brings attention to the themes and needs of any planet, sign, or house it passes over. For example, if your natal Mars is in Capricorn, you may notice when the Sun makes its yearly trip through Capricorn that the themes and body areas of your natal Mars become more prominent. If this is the case, you could use the information in both the Capricorn and Mars sections to adjust your personal care.

Keep in mind that sunlight can be extreme. Sunburns, glares, heatstroke, and being blinded by its brightness are some examples. In astrology, the Sun is not a disease-inflicting planet, but occasionally when the Sun is unhealthy, or it's being afflicted by another planet, it may contribute to our blind spots, inner biases, and things we'd rather not see.

If you're in a time of maintaining good health, I encourage you to use the transiting Sun (the Sun in today's sky) as a body-care clock, as discussed in chapter 2.

SUN FOODS: LEO

Nutrients: vitamin D, vitamin A, magnesium, iodine

Most of these foods belong to the Sun because of their color and how or where they grow. They may be yellow or orange, require full sunlight, grow in a hot or tropical climate, or on a vine. They may have the word *sun* in their name, are dried by the sun, have a bright flavor, or are good sources of the Sun's nutrients. Some Sun foods have a connection with royalty. They may be decadent, eye-pleasing, and aromatic.

Vegetables and Fruit	Grains, Beans, and Legumes	Nuts and Seeds	Culinary Herbs and Spices	Meat and Seafood	Fats and Oils	Sweeteners	Possible Allergens or Trouble Foods*
Bananas	Corn	Almonds	Bay leaves	Beef	Coconut oil	Blackstrap molasses	Cane sugar, sucrose
Bell peppers (yellow, orange)	Peanuts	Sunflower seeds	Lemongrass	Chicken	Olive oil	Cane sugar	Casein
Carrots	Rice (all variations)	Walnuts	Lovage	Goat		Coconut sugar	Chocolate
Citrus			Mustard	Lamb			Citrus
Coconut			Nutmeg				Corn
Dried fruit (especially dates, raisins)			Peppermint				Egg yolks
Figs			Rosemary				Peanuts
Grapes			Saffron				Tomatoes
Mangoes			Tarragon				
Olives			Turmeric				
Plantains							
Pomegranates							
Sunchokes							
Sweet potatoes							
Tomatoes							

* Any of the foods listed in this chart may become problematic in the right astrological context, but these are the most likely Sun aggravators.

MOON
Nourishing

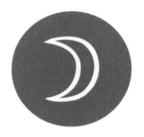

The Moon is like a satellite dish, picking up cosmic information emitted by all the planets and beaming it down to us. The Moon receives and delivers the Sun's vital energy to all the cells of the body. It's the primary planet in energy level and digestion.

Moon Basics

Rules: Cancer

Element: Water

Qualities: Cold, moist

Key Action: Reflecting, circulating, receiving, reacting, nourishing

Body Functions: Body rhythms (appetite, circadian rhythm, energy flow, menstrual cycle), nourishment habits and digestion, emoting, pregnancy, lactation, fluid motion and secretion (blood, lymph, water)

Lunar Imbalances

Deficiency Not Receptive Enough	Shared	Excess Too Receptive
Dryness, dehydration Fertility, pregnancy, and lactation challenges Insomnia Rejection of nourishment: eating disorders, ignoring body signals, poor appetite, vomiting	Functional and emotional digestive issues Inconsistent daily energy Psychosomatic conditions	Excess dampness harboring fungus, yeast, bacteria, or worms Extreme moodiness Fluid retention, stagnation, swelling, and phlegm Somnolence Weepiness

Planetary Balancing

STRENGTHEN WITH

More Moon

Your Moon sign or the current Moon sign

BALANCE WITH

Mars enlivens a sleepy Moon.

Saturn stabilizes and dries an inconsistent, boggy Moon.

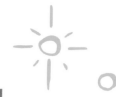

Lunar Food and Movement

Although the Moon has a few of its own correlations, it's mostly just a reflector. It magnifies the food and movement needs of whatever zodiac sign it's in or planet it's near. But very generally, when the Moon is sick, it needs to be rested and comforted. *How* it needs to be soothed will depend on where it is in your natal chart or in today's sky. The best way to care for your natal Moon or today's Moon is to use the self-care information in the corresponding sign section.

Moon food is gentle on the tummy and the heart. It's the same with exercise. On its own, the Moon doesn't have a natural affinity for vigorous movement. It's watery, sleepy, and more interested in body restoration. When the Moon needs some attention, take extra time off, receive bodywork, take a bath, do some gentle stretching, or just do some intuitive movement. Do what feels good and nourishing.

As the Moon rotates around your birth chart each month, it activates each planet, sign, and house. As this occurs, you may notice changes in appetite, energy level, metabolism, and mood. For example, when the Moon activates your natal Mars, you may experience more hunger, liveliness, or irritation; when the Moon activates your natal Saturn, you may experience lower appetite and a more serious mood. I encourage you to keep a lunar symptom journal to discover your monthly patterns.

The Sun and Moon are the foundations of astrological movement as discussed in chapter 2.

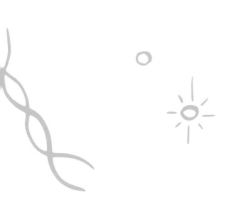

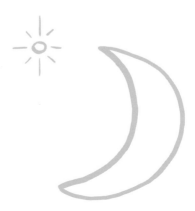

MOON FOODS: CANCER

Nutrients: general ruler of water-soluble vitamins, riboflavin (B2), potassium

The Moon has an affinity for cool, water-rich foods that are creamy and sweet or rather bland. They may grow in damp environments, swim in the sea, or have *water* in the name. The Moon rules most green foods, including crisp lettuces and other leafy greens. Lunar dishes are often comforting. Soups, stews, casseroles, and cherished family recipes are very lunar. Foods high in the Moon's nutrients are also nourishing for this planet.

Vegetables and Fruit	Nuts and Seeds	Culinary Herbs and Spices	Meat and Seafood	Dairy and Eggs	Fats and Oils	Possible Allergens or Trouble Foods*
Bok choi	General ruler of all seeds	Purslane	General ruler of all seafood	All dairy and eggs generally (with Venus),	Butter	Aluminum (food additive)
Broccoli			Duck		Ghee	Cruciferous vegetables
Brussels sprouts			Goose	*especially:*		Dairy
Cabbage (all variations)			Pork	Cow's milk		Eggs
Cauliflower			Shellfish	Soft cheeses		Moldy cheese (blue cheese, brie)
Chard			Veal	Yogurt		Mycotoxins
Collard greens						Nightshades
Cucumbers						Shellfish
Jicama						Water impurities
Kale						Yeast
Lettuce						
Melons						
Mushrooms						
Okra						
Peaches						
Pumpkins						
Sea vegetables (kelp, nori, wakame, etc.)						
Spinach						
Squashes (all variations)						
Sweet potatoes						
Truffles						
Water chestnuts						
Watercress						
Zucchini						

* Any of the foods listed in this chart may become problematic in the right astrological context, but these are the most likely Moon aggravators.

MERCURY
Connecting

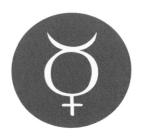

Mercury is the planet of connecting. It sends, carries, and receives information and connects one organ system to another. Mercury imbalances tend to coincide with extremely busy, high-stress times or the periods of exhaustion following them. When Mercury is off, biological information can feel unnecessarily complicated or incomplete, missing vital steps and details.

Mercury Basics

Rules: Gemini, Virgo

Element: Earth

Qualities: Cold, dry

Key Action: Connecting

Body Functions: Nervous, respiratory, hormonal

Mercury Imbalances

Deficient Too Slow	Shared	Excess Too Fast
Brain fog, poor cognition and memory Caffeine dependency Depression Poor coordination, slow reaction times, clumsiness Respiratory vulnerability Sensitivity to light and sound Social isolation: self-imposed or other	Headache Low stress tolerance Nervousness Overwhelm Poor breathing	Accident prone Anxiety Caffeine sensitivity Compulsive device checking High strung Insomnia Jumpiness Muscle spasms and cramps Nerve pain Panic attacks

Planetary Balancing

STRENGTHEN WITH

More Mercury

Gemini or Virgo

BALANCE WITH

Jupiter expands a detailed Mercury.

Venus calms a wound-up Mercury.

Saturn anchors a spacey Mercury.

Neptune sedates an anxious Mercury.

Feeding a Deficient Mercury

When Mercury is deficient, small decisions such as what to eat can leave you staring in the fridge blankly. It may feel counterintuitive, but surrendering and allowing Mercury to be slow and adjusting your lifestyle to match will get you back up to speed faster. Slow Mercury times go against the expectations of modern culture, and this is usually what's causing us the most pain.

When Mercury is deficient, it needs more time to process everything, including food. We can support this by simplifying meals. Our intention becomes bringing clarity and brightness to the mind in as few steps as possible. Seasons of Mercury deficiency are not the times for elaborate recipes and long ingredient lists. Give yourself a protein, a vegetable, a starch, and a fat at each meal. Use plain and easy prep methods and don't worry yourself with herbs and spices beyond salt and pepper. This may feel bland at first, but it gives Mercury a much-needed complexity break. Gut discomfort commonly pops up during these times and an added plus of eating simply is being able to pinpoint food reactions with much more clarity. Another benefit of simplifying and slowing down is that it frees up more mental space for us to notice and adjust our self-talk around food, which is one of Mercury's functions.

A deficient Mercury can feel burdened, and we want to help it feel more buoyant. The great nutrition debate always seems to center around carbs versus fat for fuel. But in astro-nutrition, we try to understand that all foods serve a purpose depending on the chart in front of us and the sky above us. Deficient Mercury often needs quick-energy foods that are light and easy to break down. This could mean simple, single-ingredient foods such as white rice, steamed vegetables, potatoes, squash, or fruit.

It may be tempting to reconstruct your entire diet and do something dramatic to wake up Mercury, but it's likely you don't have all the info you need right now to make an accurate choice or the brainpower to support it long term. Instead of reaching outward for more info to process, give yourself less. Mercury deficiency times often end with eureka moments, but they never come through reaching. This is a great opportunity to shut out the noise, go inward, and reconnect with your inner food knowing.

MERCURY FOODS: GEMINI, VIRGO

Nutrients: Thiamine (vitamin B₁)

Mercury and its signs live for details, and we see this mirrored in their corresponding foods. Mercury foods, such as beans and grains, come in a great number of pieces or have tons of seeds. They may grow in clusters or be gathered in bunches. We see detailed and curious Mercury in wispy herbs such as dill and the feathery tops of carrots and fennel. Whether plant or animal, these foods are energetically light.

Vegetables and Fruit	Grains, Beans, and Legumes*	Nuts and Seeds	Culinary Herbs and Spices	Meat and Seafood	Sweeteners	Possible Allergens or Trouble Foods**
Bananas	General ruler of grains, beans, and legumes	Hazelnuts	Aniseed	Chicken	All raw or minimally refined sugars (turbinado, Sucanat, etc.)	Beans
Berries		Hemp seeds	Caraway seed	Game birds		Caffeine
Carrots		Walnuts	Chervil	Turkey		Corn
Celery	Amaranth		Dill		Honey	Gluten
Endive	Barley		Fennel seed			Grains (especially wheat)
Fennel bulb	Buckwheat		Fenugreek			
Mushrooms	Bulgur		Licorice			
Pomegranates	Corn		Marjoram			
Turnips	Couscous		Oregano			
Zucchini	Lentils		Parsley			
	Millet		Sorrel			
	Oats		Star anise			
	Quinoa		Tarragon			
	Rice (especially brown and wild)					
	Spelt					
	Wheat					

* It's important to note that one grain or bean may be intolerable for Mercury, while many others are just fine and even healing. Don't rule out the entire food group. It's more often a case-by-case basis.

** Any of the foods listed above may become problematic in the right astrological context, but these are the most likely Mercury aggravators.

Feeding an Excess Mercury

When Mercury is excess, we may experience a temporary boost in metabolic rate and require more calories or more frequent food. Snacking and food timing are a hot nutritional topic, but from an astrological perspective, these short periods of Mercury excess often feel more comfortable with consistent fuel. But regardless of when we're getting calories, we want to supply them in a way that's anchoring and dense.

Instead of adding to Mercury's sense of urgency, we want to incorporate foods that bring a calm alertness to the nervous system. Both excess and deficient Mercury need high-quality protein for neurotransmitter health, but excess Mercury may need more fat, like a weighted blanket for anxiety. Supporting Mercury with regular mealtimes, protein, fat, and root vegetables allows it to not just have ideas but to do something useful with them. If excess Mercury doesn't receive the nutrition it needs, it's likely to just keep running in circles, cogitating for nothing.

The most important thing we can do is to slow down to eat. When Mercury's in a rushed state, it's easy for digestive steps to be skipped. Swap out meals in front of a screen for real human conversation. And although slowing down is ideal, sometimes we just need to take our nutrition on the go. Traditionally, Mercury rules foods that come in pods. If we expand and modernize this idea, that includes conveniently packaged foods that are ready-made and easy to carry. I prefer homemade food, but when you're in a Mercury pinch, you may need to grab takeout or a protein bar. And if you're going to have caffeine, try to weigh it down by consuming it at meals or with a fat source.

Movement for Deficient Mercury

When Mercury is deficient, our desire to move may feel nonexistent. It's typical to feel uncoordinated or to reach fatigue more quickly compared to just a few weeks ago. During this time, we want to give Mercury plenty of space to recoup, without surrendering to stillness. There are *certainly* times where complete stillness is necessary, but moving is what Mercury does. Even in states of deficiency, movement tends to make Mercury feel instantly better.

To help Mercury get moving, make things ridiculously simple. Give Mercury clear directions. Know exactly what workout you're going to do before you do it. Know exactly what you're going to wear and set it out the night before. If food is a barrier, plan and know exactly what you're going to eat before or after your workout to free up mental space. These things may seem silly, but they're a lifeline when Mercury is troubled.

Keep movement simple. When you don't have a ton of motivation and brainpower, it's best to just stick to the basics. This means minimal equipment, minimal number of exercises, simpler workout structures, and swapping any complex movements for foundational patterns. Instead of running all over the gym, choose one or two tools to work with. Just like reducing the number of meal ingredients, keep the list of exercises per workout succinct. Mercury's ability to process is reduced and we don't want to add to the backup. Five exercises or less is my personal preference.

If your main form of exercise is yoga or group classes, the same simpli-fication suggestion applies. This could take many forms, but one example is focusing solely on one type of practice, such as moderate hatha yoga or restorative classes, instead of sampling everything the studio has to offer. Sure, you're not in charge of the exercises the instructor calls out, but you can pick and choose which classes you go to and how many. Less is usually more during times of Mercury deficiency.

You may also need to lower your overall workout intensity. During Mercury deficiency, exercise ideally supports your mental health and helps you stay alert throughout the day. Further exhausting the central nervous system by constantly bringing yourself to your threshold is the opposite of what you want to do. You don't have to completely remove high-intensity exercise, just give it some limits. One short high-intensity session per week is plenty for deficient Mercury, *maybe* two, if you're used to high exercise output. I feel very energized by hard conditioning work, but I might limit it to five minutes at the end of a session a few times per week.

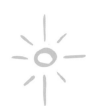

Movement for Excess Mercury

When Mercury is excess, the nervous system is heavily activated and we may feel wired and jumpy. Most of the time, I want to match Mercury's vibe and give it a vigorous exercise outlet so that it doesn't express worry and anxiety in my mind, body, or life. If Mercury is going to be restless, I like to give it something constructive to do.

You may feel like increasing your overall workout intensity and frequency during this time. Remember that Mercury is a respiratory planet. When it's anxious or squeezed, you want to give it as much oxygen as possible. This Mercury needs to breathe, and you can help it by working on your aerobic capacity. But don't hop straight on the treadmill. Excess Mercury has a short attention span and wouldn't be caught dead doing long, slow distance. Try hill repeats, stair work, sprints, or put your strength training into a Mercury-friendly interval format to keep things quick. Head to a dance class, step aerobics, or anything else that requires coordination and is fast paced and mentally stimulating. You can also engage Mercury by doing your workout at a different time, in a different place; doing your normal routine backward; trying a new class; or picking up a new piece of equipment. Mercury is the planet of travel and likes to cover some ground. Even if it's outside of your norm, you may crave running, cycling, or walking during this transit.

If Mercury is moving too fast and about to go off the rails, bring in a few movement controls. Place high-intensity movement early in the day to keep it from disrupting sleep. Take inventory of your training program and make sure it has a clear purpose and progression. Things can be fun, fast, and variable and still be structured. Program and class hopping are okay for a short Mercury transit, but if you allow yourself to just do random exercise for too long, you're not supporting Mercury long term.

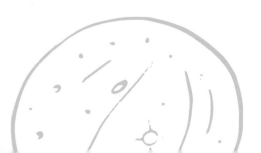

VENUS
Softening

Venus's job is to maintain body harmony and homeostasis. We tend to take this function for granted while Venus tirelessly delegates this hormonal balancing act behind the scenes. When Venus is sick, we may experience a combination of hormonal instability and feeling physically heartbroken or grieved.

Venus Basics

Rules: Taurus, Libra

Element: Water (varies among some traditions)

Qualities: Moist, cooler or warmer depending on placement

Key Action: Softening, relating

Body Functions: Homeostatic, hormonal, renal, circulatory (venous)

Venus Imbalances

Deficient Too Dry	Shared	Excess Too Wet
Amenorrhea, scanty menses Brittle hair or nails Difficulty receiving love, help, compliments, gifts Dry skin Frequent, scanty, or painful urination Infertility, miscarriage Low libido Neglecting basic self-care Vaginal dryness	Irregular menses Hormone-related skin changes Negative self-talk PMS Poor circulation, varicose veins, spider veins, blood clots Reproductive hormone imbalances	Confusing manipulation, control, and demand as love Elevated blood glucose, diabetes Fungal or yeast infections Hormonal acne Premenstrual dysphoric disorder (PMDD), heavy menstrual bleeding, uterine fibroids, leucorrhea, ovarian cysts, cystic or tender breasts Water retention, edema, swelling Weepiness, crying fits

Planetary Balancing

STRENGTHEN WITH

More Venus

Taurus and Libra

BALANCE WITH

Mars tones a lazy Venus.

Mercury quickens a sluggish Venus.

Saturn dries, disciplines, and gives Venus structure.

Uranus shakes up a sleepy or bored Venus.

Feeding a Deficient Venus

Feeding a deficient Venus is less about nutrition science and more about heart-centered food. This Venus is brittle and fearful, and it chronically braces itself for the next hurt on the horizon. During Venus healing, we want our food to create a feeling of trust and belonging that allows the energetic heart to soften and relax. Venus uses food as a mirror for self-worth. Every meal becomes an opportunity to mirror back to ourselves how incredibly valuable and precious we are, even if we don't feel it yet.

To understand the energy of a heart-centered meal, think about what a parent might feed their sick child or what you might serve someone you love when they're grieving. In times of Venus deficiency, it's our turn to take the role of responsible heart-tender in our own lives. Venus meals soothe, nourish, and mend. They're subtle, centering, and, yes, sweet in flavor, but not always in the popular sense of the word.

Desserts and treats certainly belong to Venus, and they have a role to play in Venus healing, but they aren't therapeutic-grade Venusian food. The medicinal sweetness we need during this time is found in complex carbohydrates such as starchy vegetables, legumes, grains, and fruit. Sweet is associated with Venus because it's harmonizing. It relaxes, soothes, and fills both the heart and the tissues. Many sweet foods are also moistening and help refresh the body fluids, something this dry Venus often needs help with. Moisture allows things to mix and merge, and when Venus is withered, we can use dietary moisture to help it reconnect both physically and emotionally.

During times of Venus deficiency, we also want to keep our food relatively neutral. Since our goal is to harmonize, aggressive food flavors, temperatures, or amounts entering the system may feel disruptive.

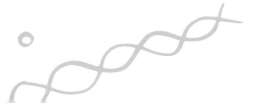

Feeding an Excess Venus

An excess Venus is typically so damp that it experiences pathological mixing and merging. This Venus may have trouble maintaining a separate self and could find itself in codependent relationships, manipulating or being manipulated, or experiencing obsession and dramatic outbursts. Physically, excess moisture can become a welcome home for unwanted bacteria, fungi, parasites, or waste. We can address pathological dampness, both physical and emotional, nutritionally. Whether Venus is experiencing insulin resistance, dealing with severe PMS, has a fungal overgrowth, or all three, we need to focus on balancing blood sugar, reducing dampness, optimizing the gut-hormone relationship, and eliminating waste.

Traditional Venusian nutrition is sweet and rather carbohydrate rich, aiming to create a cozy feeling of heaviness. But when Venus is waterlogged, adding more of these qualities to the body may make things worse. If that's the case, bring in opposing planetary food forces to lighten things up. A Saturn or Mars approach to nutrition may feel more appropriate for an excess Venus. Saturn nutrition can dry up and discipline an unruly Venus, while Mars nutrition can warm and invigorate it. The stars of a Venus excess plate are protein and foods that drain dampness. Dark leafy greens bring an energetic lightness to the body and their bitter flavor dries up Venus. Other foods that dry dampness include algae, asparagus, celery, seaweed, turnip, vinegars, and other foods that are bitter or aromatic.

To help Venus regulate its fluid balance, we also need to strengthen the kidneys. But because Venus is the regulating planet of the body, it doesn't respond positively to extremes. It responds to tenderness. Intense kidney flushes or cleanses aren't recommended. The best way to support the kidneys during a Venus imbalance is to hydrate, manage blood sugar, lower toxic exposure in daily life, and address the emotional and relational triggers at the root of Venus's illness.

VENUS FOODS: TAURUS, LIBRA

Nutrients: Carbohydrates, vitamin E, niacin (vitamin B₃), copper

Venus foods are colorful and fragrant. Most are sweet, juicy, and may conjure images of love or sex. Desserts, confections, pastries, and beautiful arrangements of any food belong to this decadent planet. Venus is the general ruler of all sugar and fruit, and it shares dairy and eggs with the Moon. It also shares many legumes with Mercury, but Venus's tend to be fleshier, larger, and green or white in color. If you love to eat it, it probably belongs to Venus.

Vegetables and Fruit	Grains, Beans, and Legumes	Nuts and Seeds	Culinary Herbs and Spices	Meat and Seafood	Dairy and Eggs	Fats and Oils	Sweeteners	Other	Possible Allergens or Trouble Foods*
General ruler of all fruit, especially stone fruit	General ruler (with Mercury) of beans and legumes	Chestnuts	Basil	Beef	General ruler (with the Moon) of dairy and eggs	Butter	General ruler of all sugar, especially fruit sugars	Aphrodisiacs	Dairy
Apples	Chickpeas	Walnuts	Cilantro	Chicken			Date sugar	Chocolate	Eggs
Apricots	Fava beans		Cloves	Kidney organ meat			Honey	Wine	Fruit sugar/fructose
Artichokes	Green beans		Fennel	Oysters					Gluten
Asparagus	Green peas		Marshmallow	Veal					Soy
Avocados	Kidney beans		Mints	Venison					
Berries	Lentils		Oregano						
Cherries	Lima beans		Parsley						
Dates	Rye		Sorrel						
Figs	Soybeans		Thyme						
Grapes	Wheat		Vanilla						
Mangoes	White beans (cannellini, great northern, navy)								
Nectarines									
Olives									
Parsnips									
Peaches									
Pears									
Plums									
Sweet potatoes									
Tomatoes									

* Any of the foods listed in this chart may become problematic in the right astrological context, but these are the most likely Venus aggravators.

Movement for Deficient Venus

When Venus is weakened, we can soften the edges of our movement practice and shift the focus from effectiveness or performance to simply feeling good. Deficient Venus needs movement to be a pleasant, balancing experience that leaves it feeling open and supported. If you can, forget about serious schedules and programs and allow movement to be heart-reviving.

When Venus is weary, you may feel like lowering overall workout intensity. Venus's homeostatic mechanism is weak, which makes it easy to overtax the body and delay healing. Avoid revving the heart rate to an extreme. When Venus can't balance itself, high highs later lead to low lows. But moderate cardio is very medicinal for a depressed Venus because it lifts the spirit and comfortably opens the lungs, moving grief through the body in a way that feels safe.

Deficient Venus is already emotionally and physically dry, so we don't want to sweat too much. Instead, we can use movement to rebuild the tissues and hydrate the body. This can be physical or symbolic. Connecting with others during movement, incorporating more flexibility into your routine, exercising in water, or simply giving yourself enough space to make intuitive changes as you're working out are all ways to give Venus some juice.

Times of Venus deficiency often coincide with seasons of repairing or adjusting our relationship with beauty and pleasure. For many, simply taking movement outside and communing with nature is enough, but also be mindful of your greater movement environment. Moderate what music you listen to, what images you see, body self-talk, and even what clothing you wear. Inquire how these things are reflecting and encouraging a higher relationship with beauty, value, and self-worth.

Movement for Excess Venus

When Venus is in excess, it's almost too damp to function optimally. In movement, when we want to dry up Venus, the first thing to come to mind is sweating. The amount we sweat varies greatly depending on external and internal factors, and it's *not* a measurement of workout "success." But in a time like this, safely encouraging excess water to leave the body may feel supportive. In some cases, an excess Venus will have trouble getting a sweat going and may need to play with variables such as hydration, clothing, room temperature, and increased intensity.

Excess Venus needs a strong emotional outlet, and high-intensity exercise can become a medicinal channel. Also medicinal is dance or movement in studios with a striking ambience. But because any excess planet can become dependent on high-intensity emotional or physical states, it's important to monitor high-intensity exercise. Swapping one for the other will not solve the underlying problem. Instead, the overall training approach needs to have a healthy balance of high-intensity bursts and structural support, usually accomplished through strength work. Symbolically, this gives Venus the opportunity to express intensity and feel deeply while also learning how to bring itself back to baseline and not get lost in the drama. It's also important that Venus finds other emotional outlets and care strategies beyond exercise.

On the other hand, Venus may feel bogged down, fatigued, and uninterested in moving. This is okay. Sometimes you just need to lean into this disinterest and rest. But also consider that this lack of interest may be due to viewing or experiencing movement as punishment. Venus is motivated by feeling good, and until Venus relates to movement as an avenue for feeling good, it's going to resist it. Once Venus reframes its movement relationship, we can bring the training tools of Saturn, Mercury, and Mars into our sessions. Time-oriented Saturn, agile Mercury, and intense Mars help give a slogging Venus a gentle kick in the pants. When Venus is in a puddle, sometimes it just needs a little structure.

MARS
Energizing

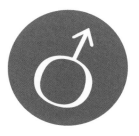

The heat of Mars wakes us up in the morning, keeps us alert, moves our muscles, and burns fuel for energy. Mars is the body's first responder and initiates both the inflammatory and immune response. When it gets orders to defend, it's going to do it no matter what, even if our own body gets damaged along the way. When Mars is dysfunctional, we stop responding to stress appropriately and the body becomes overrun with inflammation, injury, and toxicity.

Mars Basics

Rules: Aries, Scorpio

Element: Fire

Qualities: Hot, dry

Key Action: Heating

Body Functions: Metabolism (catabolic—burning up and breaking down), muscular, adrenal, protecting, inflaming, eliminating, sexual function, and arousal

Mars Imbalances

Deficient Not Strong Enough	Shared	Excess Too Strong
Anemia	Autoimmune disease	Accidents, cuts, burns, blisters, insect/animal bites and stings
Exhaustion	Chronic inflammation	Acid reflux
Loss of drive or passion	Cortisol imbalances	Acne, rashes, boils
Low blood pressure	Stress	Anaphylaxis
Low body temperature		Dehydration
Low immunity		Excessive bleeding
Low libido, sexual dysfunction		Fever and acute illness
Low stomach acid		Headache
Muscle weakness		High blood pressure
Passive-aggressive behavior		High histamine response
		Hyper-adrenaline states
		Irritability, anger, rage
		Insomnia

Planetary Balancing

STRENGTHEN WITH

More Mars

Aries and Scorpio (except for aggressive exercise if Mars is truly depleted)

BALANCE WITH

Venus calms an upset Mars.

Moon cools a hot Mars.

Saturn contains an overactive Mars.

Neptune sedates an inflamed Mars.

Feeding a Deficient Mars

When Mars is deficient, the global Fire of the body is weak and shows up most frequently as exhaustion and cortisol imbalances. The body, mind, and spirit are overloaded and simply can't receive any more stress. From a broad perspective, this means all dietary extremes are out. This is not the time to try that low-carb diet or raw food cleanse. We must relight the Fire gradually and gently to prevent aggravation, overwhelm, or relapse.

To rebuild deficient Mars, we usually need to feed it more of its associated nutrients, specifically iron, protein, vitamin B_{12}, and sometimes sodium. These nutrients are Fire generating and allow us to hold on to the Fire we have for longer. When Mars is extremely deficient, it may receive these nutrients most easily from high-quality animal sources. Although it's possible for meticulously planned vegan fare to bring Mars back to life, it's unnatural for Mars and may result in a longer healing path. In this case, you may need to leverage supplementation to ensure you're getting an adequate dose of Mars's nutrients.

Stabilizing blood sugar and getting enough protein are often pivotal during Mars deficiency. My preferred approach is to just make sure I have some protein at every feeding, whether it's a small handful of nuts or something more substantial. Although I don't encourage long-term counting of macronutrients, if you're in severe Mars exhaustion, it may be eye-opening to temporarily monitor your protein intake with the guidance of a practitioner. This will allow you to get a rough idea of your intake and decide if it might serve you to tweak it a bit as you heal.

The digestive fire may also be weak when Mars is sick. Low appetite is common, and fatigue may make skipping meals feel easier. But sharp drops in blood sugar cause Fire to flare. When there's no Fire to begin with, we end up further exhausted by the dip. Regularity not only serves a physical purpose but a psychological one. When Fire is low, we may feel betrayed by our body. To repair body trust, try to keep the same meal, sleep, and wake times every day, even on weekends. Choose something realistic because this needs to be nourishing and repeatable. Even if you don't feel hungry or tired at the appointed time, do your best to play along and go through the motions of nourishment. Eventually Mars will begin to follow this cycle on its own.

Feeding an Excess Mars

When Mars is in excess, Fire is too abundant, too hot, or burning in the wrong place at the wrong time. Instead of saving its fight for toxins and invaders, this unruly Mars also damages our body's cells and structures. This creates more waste, residue, and damage, and eventually inflammation becomes our constant state. An anti-inflammatory food approach may initially sound like a no-brainer in this case. But remember that Mars is our first responder and *anything* that causes it to hyperreact needs to be examined. Please keep in mind that the "inflamer" may not be food at all, but the food relationship, a personal relationship, disordered exercise behavior, trauma, stress, a harmful work environment, and so on. Take a critical look at the whole inflammatory picture before blaming specific foods. Mars is tricky and may set a fire in one area to distract you from the real problem. It's often easier, especially in the height of "wellness" culture, to blame an "inflammatory" food than it is to look underneath and see what really needs attention. I know from personal and professional experience that when someone is in a Mars excess (or deficient) state and they're given an overwhelming dietary protocol to follow, the stress of the experience will often drive the inflammatory cycle deeper. What we usually need to do during Mars excess is step out of this cycle completely. You may discover that a gentle, Venusian food approach feels most soothing during this time.

With that out of the way, let's talk about the possibility of inflammatory foods. First, what's inflammatory for one person may not be inflammatory for another, so use your own body wisdom as a guide. When Mars is involved, possible clues that a food (or a food thought or eating environment) may be aggravating you are hot or acute in nature, meaning they come on suddenly. Irritability, sweating, hot flashes, insomnia, headache, sharp pain, redness, itchiness, and a dramatic shift in energy level or mood are possible.

Beyond what's uniquely inflaming to you, some foods are popularly agreed upon as being inflammatory and may be wise to avoid during Mars excess depending on your personal experience. Examples are alcohol, caffeine, hydrogenated and partially hydrogenated oils (found in processed foods, margarine, canola and soybean oil), soda, sugar, and synthetic sweeteners. Depending on your presentation, this list may also include beef, citrus, commercial dairy, corn, Mars-ruled spices such as cayenne, nightshades, peanuts, pork, shellfish, sodium, soy, and wheat.

A therapeutic Mars excess plate is often colorful and full of plant foods. If Mars is extremely hot and damaging, the occasional use of raw food and vegetable and fruit juices may be indicated because they're energetically cooling. Use cooking fats such as avocado oil, coconut oil, ghee, and olive oil and inflammatory-modulating herbs and spices such as ginger and turmeric. Remember from our Mars deficiency discussion that Fire flares when blood sugar dips too low, so be sure to avoid this by prioritizing protein at every meal and not fearing carbohydrates. In Mars excess, you may find that leaner protein such as chicken, turkey, eggs, or beans and legumes feel best.

Movement for Deficient Mars

Mars deficiency often follows an immensely stressful period or any physical or psychological trauma that pushed you beyond your capacity. Movement during this time needs to be highly controlled, with the sole aim of rebuilding and restoring the body. We want to bring the Fire of Mars back to life, but it must be done very gradually, or we risk deepening exhaustion and prolonging healing.

If you haven't already, it's best to completely stop HIIT (high-intensity interval training), lengthy cardio sessions, exercise in heated rooms, and extreme anaerobic exercise where you're breathless and working near failure. These things deplete the vital fluids of the body and trigger an already worn-out Mars. Mars will use any means necessary to energize the body, and when it's in this state, it'll even break down muscle tissue to give us quick energy. This is where pain, lingering injuries, and poor muscle tone come in.

Lower the intensity, incorporate moderate resistance training, and increase calories. Swap high-intensity cardio for daily neighborhood strolls, gentle yoga, or weekend hikes. If you don't get seven to eight hours of sleep the night before, skip your training. Instead of lifting the heaviest weights or moving the fastest, work on movement quality and your body's structural integrity with isolation and balance exercises. Devote a portion of every warm-up to recruiting and activating the proper muscle fibers for the session ahead, especially the glutes. If you're a runner, taper your mileage and put a cap on

MARS FOODS: ARIES, SCORPIO

Nutrients: Protein, amino acids, fatty acids, iron, vitamin B_{12}, cobalt, folate/folic acid (vitamin B_9), sodium, phosphorus, molybdenum, selenium

Mars foods are hot, red, acidic, and distinctive in odor or taste. They're often really spicy or really bitter. People tend to love them or hate them. Or maybe you love Mars foods but they don't love you back. They may be high in protein, rich in Mars's nutrients, or mimic the warrior planet with spikes and sharp edges. Any food becomes more Mars-like when it's smoked or cooked at an extremely high temperature or over an open flame.

Vegetables and Fruit	Grains, Beans, and Legumes	Culinary Herbs and Spices	Meat and Seafood	Other	Possible Allergens or Trouble Foods*
Artichokes	Oats	All hot chilies and peppers	Red meat generally	Black tea	Acidic food
Arugula	Red beans and lentils	Basil	Hot sausages	Coffee	Caffeine
Beets		Black pepper	Lamb		Garlic
Daikon		Capers	Venison		High-sulfur foods (there are many, but alliums, cruciferous vegetables, and red meat are common triggers)
Dragon fruit		Cardamom			
Durian		Cayenne			
Eggplant		Chives			
Hot peppers		Cilantro			Hot chilies and peppers
Jackfruit		Cinnamon			Onion
Leeks		Ginger			Processed meat
Onion		Horseradish			
Passion fruit		Mace			
Pineapple		Mustard			
Radishes		Nettle			
Rhubarb		Nutmeg			
Scallions		Peppermint			
		Rosemary			
		Turmeric			

* Any of the foods listed in this chart may become problematic in the right astrological context, but these are the most likely Mars aggravators.

speed work for a bit. Skip hot yoga and vigorous flows and opt for slower, restorative practices in a warm room. If you're very depleted, it's also wise to keep your heart rate below 140 beats per minute.

Working with Mars deficiency requires us to humble ourselves and find the sweet spot where exercise is medicinal and doesn't contribute to depletion. Ensure you're working in your sweet spot by implementing a few check-ins after training. Notice how you feel immediately afterward, then six, twelve, twenty-four, and forty-eight hours afterward. If any of your Mars deficiency symptoms worsen during this time, it's a clue that you need to back off even more. If you take this opportunity to heal seriously and give Mars what it needs, it often responds very quickly.

Movement for Excess Mars

In Mars excess, we're riding a fine line between high output and exhaustion. We have a unique opportunity to pump the brakes, put in some controls, and get Mars back in line. Without the controls, however, we're likely to push past the peak and dip into Mars deficiency. During these times, it's normal to feel agitated, wired, and in need of a vibrant physical outlet, but we must control the outlet so that Mars doesn't injure us along the way. Basically, we're learning how to coexist with and manage Mars's Fire so that we don't get burned.

If you're very active, it may be helpful during this time to create a clear mental distinction between regular exercise and challenge days. There's a specific time and place for warrior-like output, but it should be limited to once or twice per week. The rest of the week should be focused on strength, skill, and balancing the body's structure. This way, when we show up for our harder workouts, we'll have the fuel necessary to get them done instead of coming in prefatigued.

We also want to engage with more intelligent forms of intensity. Instead of overloading on HIIT, teach yourself to do repeatable, high-quality work. This requires appropriate pacing and rest intervals. For example, let's say you have a challenging circuit of exercises that you want to repeat five times. Unwise Mars would do this as fast as possible with minimal rest, getting slower and sloppier each round. This will feel as though you're working hard, but it's inefficient and not doing you any favors. Instead, coach yourself to work at

85 percent effort and take two to three minutes between rounds. Rather than racing through the circuit, aim to finish each round in the same amount of time. It'll get progressively harder, but if you're truly pacing yourself, it should be sustainable.

Sometimes, excess Mars desires to feel out of breath more frequently. Give Mars what it wants but stay in the safe zone by limiting truly high-intensity work to ten minutes or less. Mars loves a battle, and you may find signing up for a race or competition to be a helpful outlet as well. It's also important to diversify your stress relief tool kit. If your only form of stress relief is to work out harder, Mars excess is going to push you beyond the edge. Find other outlets that allow you to express Mars energy beyond sweating.

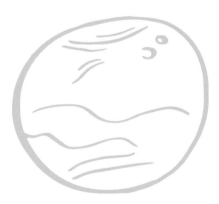

JUPITER
Satisfying

Jupiter represents bounty, plenty, and expansion in astrology. Its physical functions are to grow, regenerate, and store. As with every other planetary function, these are necessary for good health, but problems arise when Jupiter grows too much or stores too much, or perhaps not enough. Although Jupiter is largely considered a benefic planet, its diseases are some of our most common modern-day ailments.

Jupiter Basics

Rules: Sagittarius, Pisces

Element: Air

Qualities: Hot, moist

Key Action: Growing, expanding, inflating, supporting, filling, storing

Body Functions: Liver function, pituitary gland function, arterial circulation, left brain function

Jupiter Imbalances

Deficiency Deflated	Shared	Excess Too Inflated
Blood deficiency	Blood and clotting disorders	Fatty liver disease
Depression	Blood sugar dysregulation	Fluid retention, edema
Fat malabsorption	Circulatory problems	Growths, cysts, boils, enlargements, and tumors
Hypoglycemia	Gas and bloating	Hyperglycemia
Lung weakness	Pituitary gland disorders	High cholesterol
Poor liver function		Too much of anything (blood sugar, energy, fluid, hormone)
Poor memory		

Planetary Balancing

STRENGTHEN WITH

More Jupiter

Sagittarius and Pisces

BALANCE WITH

Mercury focuses an overexuberant Jupiter.

Saturn anchors a floating and excessive Jupiter.

Jupiter Nutrition

Jupiter desires to expand. This isn't a cute idea; it's a basic survival need. If Jupiter is deprived and not allowed to expand, explore, and enjoy life, it will experience intense and uncomfortable craving. Craving will drive Jupiter to meet its needs in any way possible. It's commonplace in astrology to equate Jupiter with "over-" anything: overeating, overworking, overconsuming, overspending. Sure, this may be something Jupiter acts out with. But we must look at *why* these things are happening. Over is usually a response to under. It's a signal that a need is not being met. Meeting Jupiter's needs creates satiation and stops the cycle of craving. Jupiter transits are opportunities to acknowledge your needs, meet them compassionately, and cultivate an experience of satisfaction.

Within food, cultivating satisfaction might mean allowing yourself to eat what you want, or using delicious, rich ingredients. By the way—Jupiter is the ruler of dietary fat. Butter, cheese, wine, steak, bacon, and creamy sauces tend to get Jupiter salivating. But cultivating satisfaction also includes realizing when a certain need isn't met by food and giving it what it actually requires. Cultivating satisfaction may also include examining the subtle conditions you've put on your food choices. Most people I see vehemently deny operating from a diet mentality, but with closer inspection, we often uncover food conditions like, "I can eat this, but I can only have a couple bites." Or, "I can eat that if I go on a run tomorrow." These subtle rules make Jupiter feel limited and often cause it to lash out later. Keep in mind too that sometimes what you may register as a "craving" is actually motivated by a physiological need, such as a nutrient deficiency.

We've been conditioned through societal and media messaging that we can't be trusted to eat what we want. And when exploring the concept of satisfaction with clients, I'm often met with a lot of fear and skepticism. But here's the thing—Jupiter is a life-preserving planet. Its job is to heal and regenerate the body and promote well-being. If Jupiter is trusted with food and allowed to *mindfully* explore satiation, it will choose foods that increase its physical, mental, and emotional experience of health. Expansion is not synonymous with out-of-control behaviors, eating or other. A loss of control doesn't feel satisfying. Satisfaction also extends beyond taste. It includes how you feel after eating. Do you like the way you feel? Do you feel energized? Do you feel supported in the hours after eating? If I eat something that tastes delicious but have terrible stomach pain afterward, this isn't a fully satisfying experience, and I may not choose to eat that food again. This is because my definition of satisfaction includes feeling good.

From a medical nutrition therapy perspective, another way Jupiter may love to expand is by filling the belly with air. Gas, belching, and bloating are common Jupiter-related complaints. Jupiter transits may influence us to eat too fast, which can contribute to bloating, but if you're chewing well and still distended, it's time to investigate. There are many underlying possibilities, but when Jupiter is involved, I'm always curious about a lack of bile, fat malabsorption, or intestine bacterial overgrowth. Remember that Jupiter rules the liver, and without proper bile production, we can't digest the healthy fats this planet needs.

JUPITER FOODS: SAGITTARIUS, PISCES

Nutrients: Fat, general ruler of fat-soluble vitamins (A, D, E, K), essential fatty acids, vitamin B_6, biotin (vitamin B_7), choline, chromium, zinc, manganese, inositol

True to form, Jupiter spans a lot of food categories. It's the ruler of dietary fat, but also shares a love of carbohydrates with Venus. Jupiter won't turn down a treat, but while Venus is sugary sweet, Jupiter generally leans toward starch. Jupiter shares many of the Moon's bland vegetables, but it'll dress them up with rich sauces. Its produce, grains, and beans are often bulbous or oversized, and anything advertised as jumbo is certainly Jupiter's.

Vegetables and Fruit	Grains, Beans, and Legumes	Nuts and Seeds	Culinary Herbs and Spices	Meat and Seafood	Fats and Oils	Sweeteners	Other	Possible Allergens or Trouble Foods*
Apples	Barley	Almonds	Aniseed	Fatty cuts of meat generally	General ruler of all fats and oils, especially saturated	Cane sugar	Alcohol and spirits	Alcohol
Apricots	Chickpeas	Cacao	Bay leaves	Poultry		Maple sugar	Chicory-based coffee substitutes	Artificial food replacements (alcohols, margarine, sugar)
Asparagus	Rice (especially short-grain, such as sushi and arborio)	Chestnuts	Chervil	Tuna and other very large fish	Butter	Maple syrup		
Brussels sprouts		Flaxseed	Cinnamon		Heavy cream			Greasy or fried food
Cabbage	Wheat	Hazelnuts	Cloves		Lard			High-FODMAP foods**
Chard		Macadamia nuts	Mace		Tallow			
Collard greens		Sesame seeds	Mints					
Dandelion greens			Nutmeg					
Endive			Sage					
Figs			Thyme					
Kale								
Leeks								
Olives								
Rutabaga								
Tomatoes								
Turnips								

* Any of the foods listed in this chart may become problematic in the right astrological context, but these are the most likely Jupiter aggravators.

** FODMAP stands for fermentable oligosaccharides, disaccharides, monosaccharides, and polyols. Common high-FODMAP foods include apples, avocados, asparagus, Brussels sprouts, cauliflower, garlic, onions, mushrooms, peas, wheat, and sugar alcohols (xylitol, erythritol, sorbitol, etc.). A low-FODMAP menu may be helpful in cases of IBS but it's a short-term solution that should be monitored and paired with other therapeutics.

Jupiter Movement

Jupiter brings a buoyant, lightheartedness to movement, but it also offers a great opportunity for physical growth. Jupiter doesn't have the serious reputation of Saturn or Mars, but it's always desiring to move beyond its current experience—to be better and achieve more. These are the qualities of a great athlete and a great workout.

We see Jupiter in the pomp, glory, and pageantry of events such as the Olympics. But for us non-Olympians, if you've ever experienced a runner's high or a moment where your soul soars during a hike or a piece of choreography, you've experienced Jupiter in motion. Anything that lifts your spirit and connects you to that ineffable vastness is Jupiter movement.

Jupiter is always pushing outward, which is why it's the ruler of arterial blood, bounding out from the heart to the tissues. Jupiter movement engorges the muscles with blood, which brings nutrients, oxygen, facilitates waste removal, and encourages muscle growth (remember that growth is Jupiter's domain). In a weightlifting context, this inflation is stimulated by something called "hypertrophy training." Instead of increasing absolute strength, this training is more about increasing muscle cell and fiber size. A very basic example is doing three sets of an exercise for eight to twelve reps. This is a classic resistance training format, but it's often done incorrectly. To trigger the right response, the weight should be heavy enough to where the last few reps are very hard and require roughly two minutes of rest between sets.

As an Air planet, Jupiter is deeply connected to breath and lung expansion. Jupiter simply needs to feel inflated, so anything that fills the muscles and lungs with oxygen makes it happy. Speaking of happiness, any movement that lightens your mood or enriches your life is Jupiter flavored. Jupiter also likes flying and being up in the air. Aerial yoga, suspension training systems, and fitness classes that prioritize jumping are often Jupiter favorites.

One Jupiter caution: sometimes this planet can leave us so optimistic or enthusiastic that we take on too much. Again, Jupiter isn't the taskmaster that Saturn is, but because it's always desiring to grow, it can lead us to naively overcommit ourselves or overdo exercise. When an overzealous Jupiter designs a training schedule, you might find yourself trying to do everything: running, lifting, dancing, yoga, and so on. Sometimes this is good medicine, but just be mindful that it's not an efficient way to get anywhere specific. A too-fervent Jupiter can eventually knock the wind out of you.

SATURN
Fortifying

Saturn has a notorious reputation in popular astrology (see the Saturn return discussion on page 218), but without it, we'd be heaps of flesh with no bones, no structure, no boundaries, and no direction. Saturn rules the tangible world that we put our trust in—a roof over our head, clothes on our back, and a job to pay the bills. Saturn gives us a foundation on which to build a healthy life. Problems occur when Saturn becomes too strong or too weak and either does its job too well or not at all.

Saturn Basics

Rules: Capricorn, Aquarius

Element: Earth

Qualities: Cold, dry

Key Action: Building, contracting, structuring, limiting, condensing, slowing, depressing, containing, solidifying, constricting, hardening, crystalizing, aging

Body Functions: Anabolism (building up); formation of bone, teeth, joints, and skin; gallbladder function, parathyroid function

Saturn Imbalances

Deficiency Creating Weakness	Shared	Excess Creating Blockage
Body wasting and atrophy	Body pain	Arthritis
Leaky gut syndrome	Bone diseases	Bone spurs, ossification
Low immunity	Chronic disease and infection	Constipation
Hypofunctioning organs or glands	Dental problems	Emotional repression
Osteoporosis, broken bones	Depression	Extremely hard on yourself
Poor emotional boundaries	Fatigue	Obstructions or blockages (bowel obstruction, lung obstruction, clots)
Severe malnutrition	Heavy metal poisoning	Stiffness and hardenings
Slow healing	Poor circulation	Stones (gallstones, kidney stones)
Structural breakdown	Skin conditions (usually dry in nature)	Toxic retention

Planetary Balancing

STRENGTHEN WITH

More Saturn

Capricorn and Aquarius

BALANCE WITH

Sun brightens a sad Saturn.

Mercury quickens a slow Saturn.

Moon softens a rigid Saturn.

Mars warms and wakes up a tired Saturn.

Venus moistens a stiff Saturn.

Jupiter expands a pessimistic Saturn.

Uranus liberates a chained Saturn.

Neptune opens a shut-down Saturn.

Saturn Nutrition

Saturn's job is to take the nutrients you've extracted from food and repair damage, build new structure, and replenish stores. If an unhealthy Saturn were to walk down the street, it might look tired and emaciated, with stooped shoulders, dry and lusterless hair, and an ashen lack of color to its face. When Saturn is pathologically active in your life, regardless of your outer appearance, the inner functioning of the body can carry this weary essence. During Saturn times, you can feel as though you simply don't have the resources you need physically, emotionally, or financially.

There are two major roots to Saturn gut issues: the actual function of the GI is hindered, or the individual is blocking their own nourishment through poor diet or severe restriction. Saturn creates functional gut issues by "drying" up the GI. There's usually a lack of all digestive secretions from top to bottom, including saliva, stomach acid, enzymes, bile, and intestinal mucus. Without these, food isn't adequately broken down and made usable, eventually leading to fatigue, pain, and nutrient deficiencies. Saturn may require digestive bitters, enzymes, sometimes hydrochloric acid, and any lacking vitamins and minerals as the underlying cause is addressed. The cold nature of Saturn also slows gut motility or motion. This may show up as chronic constipation, but it could develop into irritable bowel syndrome (IBS), small intestinal bacterial overgrowth (SIBO), or a high toxic load. This dry, cold lack of motion may play into food sensitives as well. If present, these are typically going to express as delayed hypersensitivity reactions that might not show up for many hours or even days after the food in question was eaten.

It's important to emphasize, especially when Saturn is involved, that the goal isn't to identify "bad" foods and remove them forever. The goal is to get the gut to a place where it can eat any food and break it down into its usable and unusable parts. Saturn likes rules, and once it gets into a groove of being on a super-restricted diet, it could go on forever. This may work for a while, but it'll eventually get you back to where you started—sensitivities, deficiencies, and food fear. Saturn needs a highly varied, rotating diet. If you give Saturn the same ten foods repeatedly and don't address the underlying issue, it'll develop an intolerance to those ten foods.

Saturn can make it hard to get enough calories, whether it's self-inflicted or due to illness. If you do get enough, those calories tend to lack nutrients or you may have trouble extracting them. To keep Saturn strong but supple, give it as many mineral-packed, nutrient-dense, and diverse building blocks

SATURN FOODS:
CAPRICORN, AQUARIUS

Nutrients: Protein; general ruler of minerals, vitamin C, and bioflavonoids; calcium, vitamin K, fluorine, vanadium, sulfur

Saturn food sustains us. From root vegetables to cured meat, if it can get you through the winter, it probably belongs to Saturn. Fermented, pickled, and otherwise preserved foods fall on this list not only because they last the long haul but also because of their distinctive smell. Saturn foods are the antithesis of sweet and fragrant. Their sour and bitter flavors will make you pucker. Saturn foods are energetically heavy and often black or dark in color. Fun fact: most poisons also belong to Saturn.

Vegetables and Fruit	Grains, Beans, and Legumes	Nuts and Seeds	Culinary Herbs and Spices	Meat and Seafood
General ruler of root vegetables	Barley	Black sesame seeds	Sage	Beef
Beets	Black beans	Hemp seeds	Salt of all kinds	Bison
Blackberries	Black lentils			Cured meat (bacon, pancetta, prosciutto, salami, etc.)
Black cherries	Forbidden rice			
Cassava	Fermented rice (natto)			Fermented fish
Celeriac				Mutton
Durian				
Nightshades (eggplant, peppers, tomatoes, white potatoes, etc.)				
Olives				
Onions				
Parsnips				
Potatoes and yams (all varieties)				
Pickled and fermented vegetables (kimchi, sauerkraut, etc.)				
Sea vegetables (kelp, nori, wakame, etc.)				
Spinach				

as possible. Protein is your body's builder and Saturn's official macronutrient. It's often not enough for an activated Saturn to get adequate protein; it needs optimal protein. As in Mars deficiency, if you have a Saturn-heavy chart or are undergoing a Saturn transit, you may want to explore your protein intake with a practitioner. Other Saturn tips include eating colorful food that's easy to digest. Keep the flavors simple; limit cold and raw foods; blend, mash, and puree; and focus on soups and stews.

Dairy and Eggs	Fats and Oils	Other	Possible Allergens or Trouble Foods*
Goat milk and cheese Sheep milk and cheese Stinky cheeses (blue, Camembert, brie, etc.)	Safflower oil	Bone broth and bone marrow Coffee Collagen peptides Fish sauce Gelatin, agar agar Psyllium husk Vinegars	Eggs High-oxalate foods (beets, many dark leafy greens, sweet potatoes, etc.) High-sulfur foods (alliums, cruciferous vegetables, etc.) Nightshades (eggplant, peppers, tomatoes, white potatoes, etc.) Nitrates (often found in cured meats) Shellfish Sulfites (found in fermented food, processed food, and wine, as a preservative)

* Any of the foods listed in this chart may become problematic in the right astrological context, but these are the most likely Saturn aggravators.

Saturn Movement

Saturn is a taskmaster and its vibe is heavy and laborious. It rules time and structure, and when it's healthy, it's interested in building up the body so that it can do important work. Saturn teams up with Mars to build muscle and strength, and its work takes discipline and sacrifice. Saturn is cold and slow, while Mars is hot and fast. Although both planets get major work done, they do it in different ways. Mars has an affinity for extremely high heart rates, sweating, and heaving breath. Saturn can certainly get the blood pumping, but it has an affinity for slogging, enduring experiences with no end in sight.

When working with Saturn in a gym context, you can emulate its graveness by intentionally "limiting" the body using weight, time, distance, or a mixture of all three. I highly encourage resistance training during Saturn times because this planet is quite literally resistance. Saturn routines often work with absolute strength, which requires heavy loads, lower reps, and longer recovery times between sets. But absolute strength only hits one side of Saturn. Another important part of Saturn training is strength endurance. The load is still on the heavy side but the repetition number is gruelingly high or the amount of time under tension is lengthy. Saturn works to failure. Outside of the gym, you can work with Saturn in endurance sports, especially if the terrain offers a lot of challenge.

Saturn and Neptune tend to be the most fatiguing planets, and both can coincide with lowered workout performance or desire to move. But these planets are energetic opposites. Saturn transits can most certainly correspond with illness, but unlike the diffusive and abstractly weakening force of Neptune, Saturn fatigue is generally an overworking force where external pressures steal your time and energy. Saturn transits are like an exam that lasts for a couple of years, making sure you have what it takes. It's rather standard to move in and out of more serious fatigue and experience movement restrictions or nagging injuries.

URANUS

Liberating

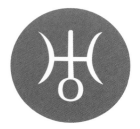

When Uranus acts on the body, things can feel unstable, buzzy, and polarized, as though your whole life is running backward or stuck in an eternal retrograde. Uranus is not subtle. Its unsmooth energy announces itself with a bang, whether in the heart, gut, energy, muscle, or mind.

Uranus Basics

Rules: Aquarius (modern)

Qualities: Whatever it wants, when and how it wants, but it tends to carry a fiery, airy, and dry imprint

Key Actions: Electrifying, firing, connecting, coordinating, pulsing, vibrating, undulating, transporting

Body Functions: Nervous and mental, thyroid function (with Mercury and Taurus), keeping body cadence and rhythms, pituitary gland function (with Jupiter)

Uranus Imbalances

Accidents, falls, breaks, tears, pulls, strains, ruptures, and bursts

Anything rare, extreme, or acute in expression

Anxiety

Conditions that swing between poles

Insomnia

Irregular body rhythms (abnormal circadian, heart, and hormonal rhythms; erratic energy levels, peristalsis, respiration, and synaptic firing)

Mental health disturbances and events

Nerve pain or degeneration

Nervous system and mental strain

Poor coordination and balance

Seizure disorders

Tics, tremors, spasms, cramps, and shooting pain in any smooth, cardiac, or skeletal muscle

Thyroid disorders

Planetary Balancing

STRENGTHEN WITH

I don't recommend strengthening Uranus, but instead soothing any other planets involved in the transit or natal configuration. In the rare case that Uranus needs strengthening, use more Uranus, Mercury, or Aquarius.

BALANCE WITH

Venus soothes a fitful Uranus.

Saturn grounds excess Uranus electricity.

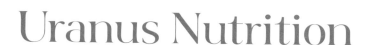

Uranus Nutrition

Uranian health is about leaving room for spontaneity but outfitting yourself with a figurative padded suit so nothing breaks along the way. Being prepared is a solid Uranus nutrition strategy. When this eccentric planet is highlighted, expect change, disruption, stress, excitement, or nervousness and try to cushion the body ahead of time. No, you never really know what the exact outcome will be, but once you get acquainted with your natal Uranus and feel a few transits to and from Uranus in real time, you'll have a pretty good idea of how and where your body processes its energy.

The most common Uranus complaint I've witnessed in practice is nervous system strain and overwhelm. The body likes regularity, and an extra helping of Uranus vibes can push the nervous system into sympathetic overdrive. Uranus excels at bringing in new ideas, breakthroughs, and solutions, but to be truly useful, its electricity must have a grounded body and mind to travel through. When Uranus is around, I want to feel like my food is reinforcing the fatty, insulating layer on my nerves, as if I could give each one a weighted blanket. Paradoxically, the more insulation we have, the faster we can receive and transmit this planet's electric brilliance. After all, transmitting nerve impulses is what these fatty layers (the myelin sheaths) do.

Exactly how we create this nutritional hug may differ for each of us, but for most people, it often means higher fat and protein intake and consuming whatever you consider to be energetically grounding food (hint: check the Capricorn and Saturn sections). It may also mean regularly timed meals, snacks, minimal caffeine, and lots of water, typically with salt or added electrolytes. It's unlikely you'll want to keep regular meals during a Uranus transit, but it'll make the experience a lot more fun and inspiring, instead of stressful. If you have a highly Uranian chart or are experiencing a major transit, waiting to eat until you feel hungry isn't always the best strategy. Uranus's mood, energy, and blood sugar swings are too quick for that. It's often best to practice preemptive nourishment.

Whatever body area Uranus is disturbing may need not only smoothing but extra nutrients. This planet can disrupt our metabolic status quo. It's as though our legs, brain, skin, or whatever body part is involved via zodiac sign is suddenly being fed erratically or not at all; its nutrient supply has been interrupted. For this reason, supplementation and a rather high, targeted intake of specific nutrients may be necessary during portions of a Uranus transit.

If Uranus's disruptions are minor and not physically serious, or if they're expressing outside of the body, give yourself permission to match its vibe nutritionally if that feels resonant. Break all your food norms. Be spontaneous. Eat the weirdest thing on the menu. Do meals backward. Completely turn your diet on its head. Whatever feels right in the moment, Uranus offers you the impetus to make it happen.

URANUS FOODS: AQUARIUS

Nutrients: None

Uranus has no traditional food rulerships of its own, but its nutritional imprint is still easy to spot. Uranus's foods will have a distinct appearance or disruptive effect. For better or worse, they tend to give you a jolt and shake up your mental state and nervous system. Perhaps they're made in a laboratory or are experimental in another way. Uranus is on the frontier of the culinary world. Any food or manner of eating that's outside of your normal consumption is Uranian for you.

Uranus Movement

Like other vibrant planets, Uranus needs an outlet. But instead of making any symptoms worse with erratic feeding patterns, you can direct Uranus's chaotic energy into something intentionally and constructively disruptive—exercise. Uranus is a natural athlete. It's explosive, fast, full of adrenaline, and comfortable with states of intensity. When your movement matches this energy, it can act as a diffuser and allow that buzzy, excess nervous energy to exit the body safely.

Uranus movement doesn't test your endurance. Uranus is shocking, not patient; so forget anything repetitive and long. Shorter, exciting routines or at least highly variable routines are preferred. During this time, movement ideally reflects Uranus's irregular essence. Put the body through bursts of activity, varying in intensity and duration. Select exercises that are explosive in nature. Anything with *jump* in its name is usually explosive, whether weighted or unweighted. Incorporate bounds, hops, drops, sprints, and speed work of all kinds. Uranus also likes weird movements. Make up some unique movement combinations, or better yet, stick to the classics and do them backward, upside down, or sideways. For example, handstand walking, backpedals, traveling kettlebell swings, and lateral box jumps. Don't get stuck doing biceps curls during a Uranus transit.

Try something new, whether it's in or out of the gym. The latest, weirdest workout craze, especially if tech is involved, has Uranus stamped all over it. I like using the "shock factor" when I'm having a Uranus transit (or Mars transit, for that matter). This isn't as scary as it sounds. For me, it might be as simple as going on a run (something I rarely do) or doing my conditioning first instead of last. Anything outside of my current movement norm will do. But if you're into catching a rush, Uranus loves extreme sports too. Final word of wisdom—Uranus blesses us with accident proneness, so make sure you're thoroughly warmed up.

NEPTUNE
Embodying

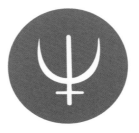

Neptune is boggy, and although it can be warm or cool, its imbalances remind me of the physical wilting and cognitive confusion brought on by an August afternoon in the deep American South. These conditions are spectral, meandering, hard to describe, and even harder to catch. Because of this, they're often misdiagnosed and go untreated or mistreated.

Neptune Basics

Rules: Pisces (modern)

Qualities: Water, humid but may be hot or cool

Key Action: Merging, sedating, calming, blending, combining, permeating, fluctuating, disintegrating

Body Functions: Pineal gland function, endorphins, cerebrospinal fluid

Neptune Imbalances

Anemia

Autoimmune conditions

Body leaking (energy, fluids, nutrients)

Body image disturbance

Chronic fatigue syndrome, post-viral fatigue

Depression

Escapism

Food, environmental, and drug allergies

Fungal infections

Hallucinations

Leaky gut syndrome, intestinal permeability

Misdiagnosed conditions

Mold toxicity, gas poisoning, other undetected poisonings

Muscle or body weakness

Mysterious infections that are confusing and changeable in nature

Organ prolapse

Psychosomatic conditions

Sleep disorders of all kinds, insomnia, narcolepsy, nightmares

Spiritually triggered illnesses

Substance use disorder

Planetary Balancing

STRENGTHEN WITH

I don't recommend strengthening Neptune, but instead stabilizing any other planets involved in the transit or natal configuration. In the rare case that Neptune needs strengthening, use more Neptune or Venus and Pisces.

BALANCE WITH

Mercury awakens a confused Neptune.

Mars pierces Neptune's fatiguing fog.

Saturn forces Neptune to embody.

Neptune Nutrition

A Neptune transit can feel a bit like a never-ending masquerade ball. "Who am I? What am I doing? How did I get here?"—these are all common Neptune questions. It can feel as if you're floating from experience to experience. And then one day, you wake up to find you're somewhere doing something you never expected or intended. Sometimes the outcome is very pleasant and better than you could've imagined (thanks, Neptune!), or perhaps it is more of a house of cards. Regardless, the road through a Neptune transit is dreamlike and slippery. Similarly, Neptune-linked nutritional issues are sneaky and not always what they appear.

Neptune has a knack for eroding structure, including physical and personal boundaries. It may allow nutrients, energy, or even a clear sense of self to leak out of the body. When Neptune is involved, you're simply more impressionable and vulnerable to external influences, whether they be a pathogen, person, or ideal. Often, Neptune food issues aren't directly food related at all. A challenging food relationship might develop in response to sustaining long-term abuse, trauma, or spiritual crisis. Or, perhaps symptoms are due to an undetected pathogenic presence, such as a chronic, low-level infection or toxic exposure. It's classic for Neptune gut problems to migrate like a fine mist and show up in a totally separate body system. Instead of crystal clear symptoms like bloating or diarrhea, you might have swelling, sinus congestion, wandering pain, water retention, dizziness, confusion, depression, or exhaustion.

Also be mindful of increased susceptibility to nutritional illusion during this time. Neptune is always seeking transcendence from suffering. And if it can't get it in a skillful way, it will get it in an unskillful way. It's common to correlate Neptune with checked-out or unconscious eating. This is possible. But it's just as possible for a Neptune-influenced person to use diet tools to distract themselves from a painful situation. This might look like getting sucked in by the shiny new wellness trend that everyone is talking about, or internalizing unrealistic beauty ideals and manipulating food in response. Or, it might just look like adopting another's food beliefs and practices as your own—without even realizing it! During Neptune times, dissociating from the body or gravitating to substances that alter the body's chemistry can feel safer or simply more attractive than attending to the difficult emotions and sensations underneath.

If Neptune is a primary health player in your chart, or if you're having a Neptune transit, chances are you're more responsive to the unseen, subtle, and chemical realms of food, specifically food energetics and alterations. By food alterations, I mean any synthetic addition or modification made to food other than cooking it. Genetically modified food falls into this category, as does highly processed food that's pumped full of dyes, flavorings, preservatives, or other chemicals or additives. If you're having mysterious digestive complaints during a Neptune transit, simply be curious about these foods.

The term *food energetics* typically refers to a food's qualities, temperature, or flavor, but with Neptune, I'm referring to your energy while eating and the energy of the food preparer, whether it's you or someone else. Food is a vessel for energy, messages, and other subtle information. When food is prepared, its energy is mixed, knowingly or unknowingly, with the energy of the preparer and consumer. During Neptune transits, we're often so attuned to energetic states outside of ourselves that if the cook is angry or depressed or if the environment is tense, that imprint has the potential, unless consciously intercepted, to travel with the food into the body. This goes for cultural food judgments and other people's food talk too. Your physical experience of a food may be completely altered depending on what you read online or what someone said to you in the breakroom at work.

But before blaming anything or anyone else, step one in Neptune health is to turn inward, check in, and develop agency where you can. Try to be more mindful of who or what is floating around in your food space and begin reclaiming it for yourself. Although it may feel safer to fly up and out, a primary part of Neptune healing is embodying and learning how to manage your own energy, feelings, and reactions. Many Neptune health issues can be markedly improved or even healed by learning this skill. This can be a complex and delicate journey, and I encourage you to seek the help of a counselor if necessary.

NEPTUNE FOODS: PISCES

Nutrients: Pantothenic acid (vitamin B$_5$)

Neptune has no traditional food rulerships of its own, but we see its watery shadow in the foods ruled by Venus and the Moon. Neptune foods may come from the sea, grow in a damp environment, or be water rich and sticky sweet. You can add alcohol, fish, mushrooms, sugar, truffles, and yeast to the Neptune list. Neptune doesn't use food to ground but to transcend and escape the confines of daily life.

Neptune Movement

Neptune movement, no matter its form, is art. Somewhat like Venus, this planet is enchanting and romantic. When Neptune is prominent in the chart or activates it by transit, we may find ourselves attracted to movement that's typically considered artistic, fluid, or form bending, such as dance, yoga, swimming, or contortion. But how we use or relate to movement can be Neptunian as well. Movement as worship, transcendence, or escape are Neptune expressions too. This is a glamorous planet, and famous or hometown star athletes may have a prominent Neptune presence as well. In the right conditions, Neptune may allow an athlete to surpass previous records or performances.

But when Neptune activates a chart by transit, the most common effects I witness are fatigue or another experience that forces someone to reorganize their relationship with exercise. Remember that Neptune transits may coincide with chronic viral, bacterial, or fungal infections, or perhaps a difficult spiritual or emotional crisis. Neptune transits may trigger a need for deep rest, or, usually toward the end of the transit, they correspond with a season of slowly reacclimating the body to exercise. This means wisely navigating post-exertional fatigue and very slowly increasing the therapeutic dose of exercise. Pathological Neptune transits are usually not the time for catabolic exercise such as running, cycling, or HIIT. The way most people use these things tears down the body instead of building it up. Instead, we need to plug the Neptune leak, slow down, and focus on building mass and structure.

If Neptune is prominent in the daily astrological weather, it's often a good time for rest, mobility and flexibility work, active recovery, or hypnotic movement of some type. This could be dance, intuitive routines, or sequences that are so fluidic you can get lost in them. By the way, intuitive routines and fluid movement aren't just things you find in dance and yoga studios. I use these techniques all the time with barbells, dumbbells, and kettlebells. Always remember that astrological exercise isn't modality specific. You can take the imprint of a planet and apply it to any movement type you choose.

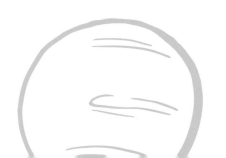

PLUTO
Surrendering

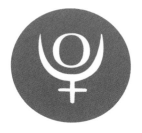

Instead of giving you a long list of hypothetical Pluto imbalances, it might be more helpful to understand that Pluto intensifies whatever it touches to a point of nonnegotiable alteration. Pluto is a midwife that carries us through all manner of births and deaths.

Pluto Basics

Rules: Scorpio (modern)

Qualities: All extremes of temperature, dryness, and moisture

Key Action: Intensifying, transforming

Body Functions: Regenerating, repairing, forming, expelling, DNA replicating and mutating

Pluto Imbalances

In my time as a medical astrologer, I've seen Pluto transits coincide with hysterectomies, gallbladder removals, and organ transplants. In each of these extreme examples, something "died" or was eliminated so that my client could literally survive or live a more pleasant life.

If Pluto acts upon your body, it'll most likely involve the parts governed by the sign it's currently in or across from, the functions of the planets it's aspecting, or the life areas of the house it's passing through. Use the suggestions in their sections to strengthen them. But unless Pluto's creating the perfect planetary alignment in your chart, it's more likely that you'll see Pluto act collectively. But you can still experience it individually. For example, I'm writing this during the COVID-19 pandemic and its fallout. This is a global Pluto experience, and it coincided with a major, once-in-a-lifetime Saturn-Pluto alignment. You may or may not have contracted the virus, but it probably changed your life in some way, directly or indirectly affecting your physical, emotional, or psychological health.

When we're collectively or personally going through a Pluto time, nourishing ourselves can feel pointless. We may tell ourselves it's selfish, small, and insignificant in comparison to the destruction and suffering we see around us or within us. We may feel confused about what nourishment even means because everything we previously believed is crumbling. But Pluto times are when being in and with our body is most vital. Like all planets, Pluto is amoral. It may trigger the karmic wave of change and bring it to the surface, but we're in charge of what newness we birth into the world. Embodied people who are compassionate, loving, and nourishing to themselves and others bring in the newness we need. By participating in personal nourishment and transformation, we make ourselves fully available as agents of global nourishment and transformation.

Pluto Nutrition

When Pluto is involved, the food experience can become very serious. For some, feeling powerless may develop into disordered eating. For others, food may be scarce and unavailable. Food could be tightly controlled as part of a treatment plan, or maybe a dietary dogma that you've clung to for years

Planetary Balancing

STRENGTHEN WITH	BALANCE WITH
I don't recommend strengthening Pluto, but instead strengthening any other planets involved in the transit or natal configuration.	The Sun helps resurrect Pluto.

is completely upended. Any food trauma we may have experienced as children is also brought to our Pluto transits. But food may or may not be the medicine Pluto is asking for. More often, Pluto "nutrition" is about surrendering, softening, and cracking open so that Pluto can do its surgery. Our food relationship is usually just an extension of the true suffering Pluto is trying to heal.

If you're undergoing a Pluto transit or if you have a strong Pluto aspect in your birth chart, I recommend focusing your nutritional approach on strengthening the planet that's being affected. For example, if Pluto is opposing your Sun, use the recommendations in your Sun sign's section. If Pluto is squaring your Venus, use the suggestions in the Venus section, or its corresponding sign section. You don't necessarily want to strengthen Pluto by eating a "Pluto diet." If Pluto made you a plate, there's a chance it could have a little poison on it—not because it wants to hurt you but because it aims to cleanse you.

You can take a kinder approach by ensuring Pluto's transformative path is clear and that the rest of your body is strong enough to support whatever work it wants to do. Removing blocks from Pluto's path may mean opening your body's detox pathways—the major ones being the skin, liver, intestines, kidneys and bladder, lungs, uterus, and nervous system. The pathways that need the most focus will be indicated by the zodiacal location of your transit. Daily elimination via sweating, deep breathing, bowel movements, high fiber, and consuming plenty of water are essential, but a more targeted approach with a practitioner may be needed occasionally.

PLUTO FOODS: SCORPIO

Nutrients: None

Pluto has no traditional food rulerships of its own, but like Mars, they'd most likely carry an extreme flavor, odor, or effect. Pluto therapeutics are intense and often applied by a licensed medical professional. Prescriptive diets used during severe illness or hospitalization are likely Pluto's. Pluto foods may help detox the body or assist in waste removal by being very fiber rich.

Pluto Movement

Just like food, Pluto movement is all about clearing the path to revolution, so don't expect it to be comfortable. Pluto movement forces you beyond your limits and isn't easily forgotten. These experiences are either short and brutally intense or long feats of endurance such as ultramarathons or events in extreme climates. In a daily fitness context, we can aid Pluto's transformation by approaching our sessions as alchemical ceremony. Bring whatever pain or poison Pluto's rooting out and surrender to the sweaty work. Approach your training like an altar and offer your movement as a spell or prayer. Pluto workouts are designed to induce catharsis. Get dirty, make noise, grunt, cry—just keep moving.

Although it waxes and wanes in intensity, a Pluto transit lasts about three years. I *don't* recommend, and you likely won't need, this type of cathartic release every day during that period. Chronic fatigue is a common Pluto symptom and you don't want to make it worse by overdoing intense exercise. Remember that Pluto doesn't just move and purge energy but also repairs and rebuilds, which require deep rest. These suggestions are for when a Pluto transit is at its peak, which is usually when it's within zero degrees of the planet it's transiting. Even that time will be quite long, so use faster astrological transits to pulse your approach. For example, ramp up your Pluto movement when the Moon passes by Pluto in the sky, or if the Sun, Mercury, Venus, or Mars are about to zoom by.

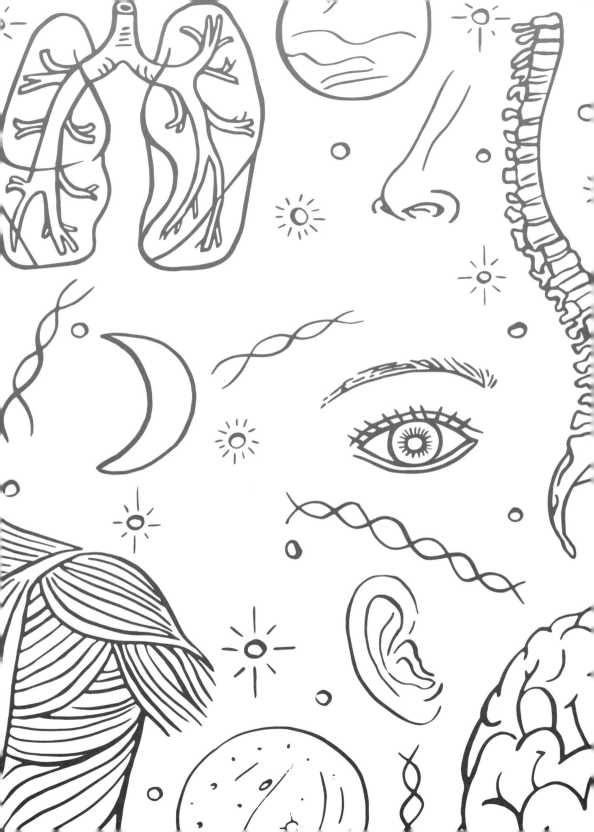

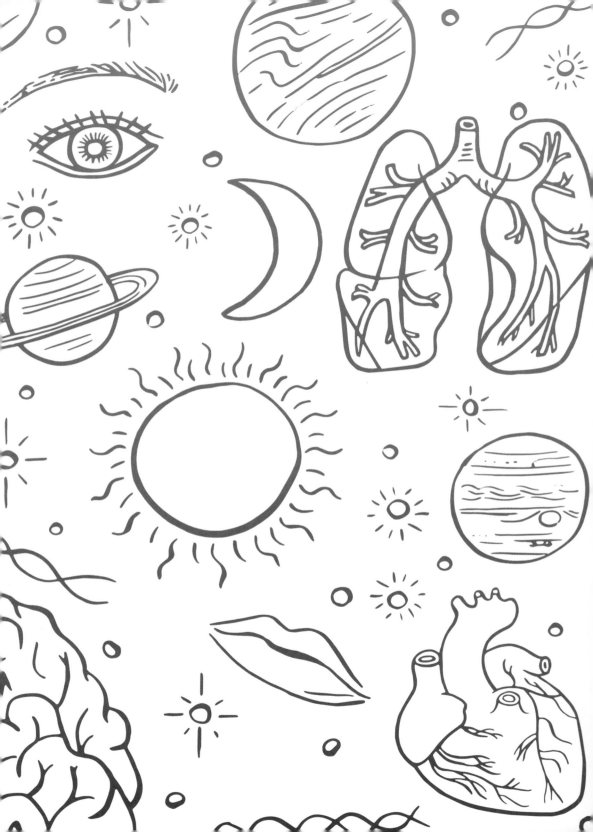

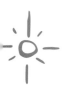
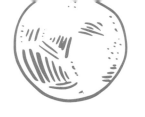

Acknowledgments

Thank you, Ryan, for the steadiest, safest, most enriching love I've ever known. You are medicine for my entire being. Thanks to my whole family for supporting me in a career I never expected to find myself in. To Momma and Sister, our chats kept me going. Dad, pencil me in for some quality lake time. Thank you, Mike and Linda, for your generosity and loving support. Nita, I love you. Thank you for always leading me back to my own authority. To my friends, especially Kelly, Renee, Islaewae, Miranda, Chelsea, Laura, Desi, and Gail—I love you. Thanks for regularly checking on me during this lonely process. Thank you, Jenn Mannhardt, for your astro-data skills.

Thank you, Roost Books and Sara Bercholz, for seeing the potential of this project and trusting me to carry it out. I couldn't have handpicked a dreamier, more compassionate group of people to work with. Big love and appreciation for my editors, Juree Sondker and Audra Figgins. Thanks also to the whole team at Roost: copyeditor Emily Wichland, proofreader Ashley Benning, indexer L. S. Summer, design director Kara Plikaitis, illustrator Caitlin Keegan, interior and cover designer Amy Sly, and the M+P team of Tori Henson and Ron Longe. Your patience, warmth, and organizing superpowers were my perfect fit.

Finally, I'm greatly indebted to the brilliant pioneers in medical astrology who directly and indirectly passed their knowledge down to me, especially Judith Hill and Andrea Gehrz. I humbly offer this to the field.

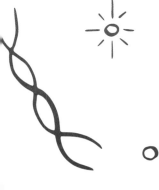

Appendix A
Symbols and Associations

MASTER LIST

Sign	Mode	Element	Ruler	Element
Aries	Cardinal	Fire	Mars	Fire
Taurus	Fixed	Earth	Venus	Water*
Gemini	Mutable	Air	Mercury	Earth*
Cancer	Cardinal	Water	Moon	Water
Leo	Fixed	Fire	Sun	Fire
Virgo	Mutable	Earth	Mercury	Earth*
Libra	Cardinal	Air	Venus	Water*
Scorpio	Fixed	Water	Mars (traditional) Pluto (modern)	Fire
Sagittarius	Mutable	Fire	Jupiter	Air
Capricorn	Cardinal	Earth	Saturn	Earth
Aquarius	Fixed	Air	Saturn (traditional) Uranus (modern)	Earth
Pisces	Mutable	Water	Jupiter (traditional) Neptune (modern)	Air

* The qualities, and therefore elements, of Mercury and Venus may change slightly depending on if they rise before or after the Sun. But for the purposes of this book, the elemental correspondences I give them here are sufficient.

GLYPH KEY

SIGNS	PLANETS & POINTS	ELEMENTS
♈ Aries	☉ Sun	△ Fire
♉ Taurus	☽ Moon	▽ Water
♊ Gemini	⊖ Rising	▽̅ Earth
♋ Cancer	☿ Mercury	△̅ Air
♌ Leo	♀ Venus	
♍ Virgo	♂ Mars	
♎ Libra	♃ Jupiter	
♏ Scorpio	♄ Saturn	
♐ Sagittarius	♅ Uranus	
♑ Capricorn	♆ Neptune	
♒ Aquarius	♇ Pluto	
♓ Pisces		

Appendix B
Symptoms

Use this appendix to identify the cosmic root of a symptom, then read the corresponding sections for guidance. Although it's certainly possible for multiple cosmic players to be involved, if several planets and signs are indicated, rely on your birth chart and intuition to determine which one feels most appropriate. For example, several planets and signs are correlated with anxiety, but there are many ways we may experience it. Does it come on suddenly with shortness of breath and a racing heart? That sounds more like Mars or Uranus. Are worrisome thoughts keeping you up at night? That sounds more like Mercury. Likewise, every sign can experience fatigue, but it may be due to different things and therefore correlated with different planets. This appendix is not exhaustive. I've only listed the most obvious correlations. In some astrological contexts, signs and planets not commonly correlated with a particular symptom may indeed be indicated.

Accidents: Mars, Mercury, Uranus, Aries, Sagittarius

Acid reflux: Mars, Cancer

Acne: Mars (red), Venus (cystic or hormonal), Capricorn, Libra, Scorpio, Taurus, sign of acne location (ex: Aries acne may be on the face, Leo on the back, etc.)

Acute onset: Mars, Uranus, cardinal signs (Aries, Cancer, Capricorn, Libra)

Addiction: Neptune, Pisces, Taurus

Allergies (environmental): Mars, Neptune, Saturn, Cancer, Gemini, Pisces, Taurus, Virgo

Anaphylaxis: Mars, Uranus, Aries

Anemia: Neptune, Saturn, Aquarius, Leo, Pisces

Anger/irritability: Mars, Aries, Scorpio

Anxiety: Mars, Mercury, Uranus, Aries, Aquarius, Gemini, Sagittarius, Virgo

Appetite change: Jupiter (increases), Mars (increases), Moon, Saturn (lowers), Cancer, Pisces, Taurus

Arthritis: Saturn, Capricorn, sign of body area involved

Asthma, shortness of breath: Mars, Mercury, Saturn, Cancer, Gemini, Pisces

Autoimmunity: Neptune, Mars, Aries, Pisces

Back pain: Mars, Saturn, Leo, Libra, Scorpio

Bites and stings: Mars, Mercury, Uranus, Pisces, Virgo, sign of bite or sting location

Bladder infection: Mars, Libra, Scorpio

Bleeding (heavy): Jupiter, Mars, Moon (menstrual), Venus (menstrual), Pisces, sign of bleeding location

Blisters and boils: Mars, Scorpio, sign of location

Bloating: Jupiter, Moon, Cancer, Pisces, Scorpio, Virgo, Air signs (Aquarius, Gemini, Libra)

Blood cholesterol (high): Jupiter, Leo, Pisces

Blood pressure (high or low): Jupiter, Mars, Aries, Aquarius, Leo, Libra, Sagittarius

Blood sugar dysregulation: Jupiter, Venus, Libra, Pisces, Taurus, Virgo

Body odor: Mars, Scorpio

Bone fracture: Saturn, Uranus, Capricorn, sign of fractured bone

Bone spur: Saturn, Capricorn, sign of spur location

Breast tenderness or swelling: Jupiter, Moon, Cancer, Venus

Brittle hair or nails: Saturn, Venus, Capricorn, Virgo

Bunions, corns: Saturn, Capricorn, Pisces

Burns: Mars, sign of burn location

Candidiasis: Neptune, Venus, Cancer, Pisces, Scorpio

Confusion: Mercury, Neptune, Sun

Congestion and phlegm: Jupiter, Moon, Venus, Cancer, Pisces, Scorpio, Taurus

Constipation: Saturn, Capricorn, Virgo, fixed signs (Aquarius, Leo, Scorpio, Taurus)

Cortisol imbalances: Mars, Aries, Libra

Cuts: Mars, sign of cut location

Cysts: Jupiter, Moon, Venus, Cancer, Pisces, Scorpio, sign of cyst location

Dehydration: Mars, Moon, Aries, Aquarius, Leo, Sagittarius

Dental problems: Mars, Saturn, Aries (upper teeth), Capricorn, Taurus (lower teeth)

Depression: Neptune, Saturn, Aquarius, Capricorn, Pisces, Scorpio

Diarrhea: Mars, Moon, Cancer, Scorpio, mutable signs (Gemini, Pisces, Sagittarius, Virgo)

Discharge: Moon, Neptune, Cancer, Scorpio, sign ruling area of discharge

Dry skin: Mercury, Saturn, Venus, Capricorn, Virgo

Dysbiosis: Jupiter, Moon, Neptune, Venus, Cancer, Pisces, Scorpio, Virgo

Ear infection: Mars, Aries, Gemini, Taurus

Eating disorders: Moon, Saturn, Uranus, Cancer, Capricorn, Scorpio, Virgo

Edema and water retention: Jupiter, Moon, Neptune, Venus, Aquarius, Water signs (Cancer, Pisces, Scorpio)

Excessive sweating: Moon, Scorpio

Fainting: Neptune, Sun, Uranus, Aquarius, Leo

Falls: Saturn, Uranus, Capricorn

Fatigue: Neptune, Saturn

Fever: Mars, Sun, Aries, Leo, Sagittarius

Food allergies/intolerances/ sensitivities: Mars, Moon, Neptune, Saturn, Cancer, Pisces, Virgo

Food poisoning: Mars, Neptune, Saturn, Cancer, Virgo

Fungal infection: Moon, Neptune, Venus, Cancer, Pisces, Scorpio

Gallstones or gallbladder pain: Saturn, Capricorn

Gas: Cancer, Jupiter, Scorpio, Virgo, Air signs (Aquarius, Gemini, Libra)

Growths and enlargements: Jupiter, sign of location

Hallucinations: Neptune, Aries, Pisces, Sagittarius

Head injury: Mars, Uranus, Aries

Headache/migraine: Mars, Mercury, Saturn, Aries

Hearing loss: Saturn, Capricorn, Gemini, Taurus

Heart palpitations: Mars, Mercury, Sun, Uranus, Aquarius, Leo

Hemorrhoids: Mars, Scorpio

Hormonal imbalances: Moon, Jupiter, Venus, Cancer, Libra, Pisces, Scorpio

Hypothermia: Saturn, Sun

Inflammation: Mars, sign of location

Insomnia: Mars, Mercury, Moon, Neptune, Uranus, Aries, Gemini, Pisces, Sagittarius

Itching: Mars, Mercury, Pisces, Virgo, sign of itchy location

Jaw pain: Aries, Taurus

Jumpiness, startling: Mercury, Uranus, Aquarius, Gemini, Virgo

Kidney stones or infection: Mars, Saturn, Libra

Lactation challenges or mastitis: Moon, Venus, Cancer

Light sensitivity: Mercury, Aries, Aquarius

Liver sluggishness, burden, or pain: Jupiter, Saturn, Virgo, Cancer, Sagittarius

Malnutrition: Moon, Saturn, Capricorn, Virgo

Memory loss: Jupiter, Mercury, Aries

Menstrual irregularities: Moon, Saturn, Uranus, Venus, Aries, Cancer, Capricorn, Libra, Scorpio

Mental-emotional disturbance (acute): Mercury, Sun, Uranus, Aries, Aquarius, Gemini, Sagittarius

Mood swings: Moon, Uranus, Aquarius, Cancer, Leo, Libra, Scorpio

Muscle spasm or cramp: Mars, Mercury, Uranus, Aquarius, sign of muscle

Muscle tear, strain, or pull: Mars, Uranus, sign of the injured muscle

Nausea: Moon, Cancer

Nerve pain, neuropathy, or neurological symptoms: Mercury, Uranus, Aries, Aquarius, Gemini, Sagittarius, sign of nerve location

Nervous exhaustion: Mars, Mercury, Saturn, Uranus, Aries, Gemini, Sagittarius, Virgo

Nervous indigestion: Mercury, Moon, Cancer, Gemini, Virgo

Nervousness: Mercury, Uranus, Gemini, Virgo

Nightmares: Neptune, Pisces

Obstructions: Saturn, sign that rules obstructed body area

Overheating: Mars, Aries, Leo, Sagittarius

Pain: Mars, Saturn, Capricorn, sign of pain location

Parasites or worms: Mars, Mercury, Moon, Neptune, Scorpio, Virgo

PMS: Moon, Venus, Cancer, Libra, Scorpio

Poor circulation: Jupiter, Saturn, Venus, Aquarius, Gemini, Leo, Libra, Pisces

Poor concentration: Mercury, Uranus, Gemini, Sagittarius

Poor coordination and balance: Mercury, Uranus, Gemini, Sagittarius

Prolapse: Neptune, Venus, sign of organ or body part involved

Psychic or spiritual attack: Neptune, Pisces

Psychosomatic symptoms: Moon, Neptune, Pisces

Rashes: Mars, Mercury, sign of rash location

Respiratory infection: Mars, Mercury, Cancer, Gemini, Pisces

Restlessness: Mars, Mercury, Uranus, Gemini, Sagittarius

Ruptures: Mars, Uranus, the sign of the body part ruptured

Sciatica: Mars, Mercury, Saturn, Libra, Sagittarius, Scorpio

Sensory overwhelm: Mercury, Uranus, Aquarius, Gemini, Virgo

Seizing, convulsing: Mercury, Uranus, Aries, Leo

Sinus issues: Aquarius, Cancer, Taurus

Skin conditions: Mars, Mercury, Saturn, Capricorn, Virgo, sign ruling skin area

Somnolence: Moon, Neptune, Cancer, Pisces

Sore throat: Mars, Taurus

Stiffness: Saturn, Aquarius, Capricorn

Stomachache: Mars, Cancer, Scorpio, Virgo

Stress: Mars, Mercury, Saturn, Uranus

Thyroid conditions: Mercury, Uranus, Taurus

Tinnitus: Mercury, Capricorn, Gemini, Taurus

Toxicity or poisoning: Mars, Neptune, Saturn

Urinary symptoms (frequent, scanty, painful, burning): Mars, Libra, Scorpio, Venus

Vision change: Moon, Sun, Aries, Aquarius

Vomiting: Mars, Moon, Uranus, Cancer

Weepiness: Moon, Venus, Cancer, Pisces

Yeast infection: Moon, Neptune, Venus, Cancer, Pisces, Scorpio

Resources

Where to Get Your Birth Chart

There are thousands of websites and apps where you can get your birth chart, but below are a few I trust. One word of professional advice: please take all computerized chart interpretations with a grain of salt.

Alabe.com

Astro.com

Astrograph.com

TimePassages App

Astrological and Lunar Calendars

Honeycomb Collective Personalized Astrological Almanac (honeycomb.co)

Magic of I Astrological Planner (magicofi.com)

Further Study

GENERAL ASTROLOGY

Books

Aspects in Astrology: A Guide to Understanding Planetary Relationships in the Horoscope by Sue Tompkins

Astrology for Yourself: How to Understand and Interpret Your Own Birth Chart by Douglas Bloch and Demetra George

Planets in Transit: Life Cycles for Living by Robert Hand

Schools

Portland School of Astrology (portlandastrology.org)

Astrology University (astrologyuniversity.com)

MEDICAL ASTROLOGY RESOURCES

My website and courses (clairegallagher.co)

Astrological Remediation: A Guide for the Modern Practitioner by Andrea L. Gehrz

A Handbook of Medical Astrology by Jane Ridder-Patrick

Medical Astrology: A Guide to Planetary Pathology by Judith Hill

Fitness

For movement demos from this book, head to clairegallagher.co/bodyastro.

EQUIPMENT

Kettlebell Kings (kettlebellkings.com)

Rep Fitness (repfitness.com)

Rogue Fitness (roguefitness.com)

Glossary

Astrology Terms

Aspects: Relationships between planets, noted by all the lines in the center of your birth chart. In medical astrology, aspects tell us how planets (a.k.a. body functions) interact with each other. There are many types of aspects, but the major aspects in medical astrology are the conjunction, opposition, square, and inconjunct.

Birth chart: Also called natal chart. A graphic representation of where all the zodiac signs and planets were at the moment of your birth. This chart takes a geocentric perspective, where you and planet Earth are at the center and the celestial bodies are orbiting around you. An accurate birth chart requires a birth date, exact birth time, and place of birth.

Degree: Each zodiac sign is made up of 30 degrees. Planets in signs have a specific degree location. For example, Saturn may be at the second degree of Aquarius.

Elements: The physical and nonphysical building blocks of the body and psyche. In medical astrology, there are four elements: Fire, Air, Earth, and Water. We have all four elements in our bodies. Elements are dynamic, and their levels naturally rise and fall, but illness occurs when one or more become excess or deficient. Each zodiac sign is associated with an element.

> **Fire signs:** Aries, Leo, and Sagittarius
>
> **Air signs:** Gemini, Libra, and Aquarius
>
> **Earth signs:** Taurus, Virgo, and Capricorn
>
> **Water signs:** Cancer, Scorpio, and Pisces

Gesture: I use the word *gesture* to describe a zodiac sign or planet's essence and how that may translate into physical needs and behavior. To grasp gesture, we tend to boil it down into keywords. But it's important to remember that signs and planets are vast bodies of energy that transcend the confines of language.

Houses: The twelve houses represent life areas (family, money, home, etc.) and may give us the context of a physical condition. Imbalances arise from, affect, or are affected by these life areas. Although any house can interplay with health, the first, sixth, eighth, and twelfth houses are directly health related. There are many house systems in astrology. I personally use and suggest whole sign houses, where one zodiac sign equals one house.

Medical astrology: An ancient branch of traditional Western astrology where the birth chart becomes a map of the body's inherent nature, workings, needs, strengths, and susceptibilities. Medical astrology may also offer guidance on the nature of an illness or disease, its root cause, and proper treatment. In this book, the terms *medical astrology*, *physical astrology*, *body astrology*, and *nutritional astrology* are used interchangeably.

Mode: How an element moves and expresses itself. Each element has multiple modes of expression. For example, Earth may come in the form of rock, soil, or plant. The three modes are cardinal, fixed, and mutable.

> **Cardinal signs:** Aries, Cancer, Libra, and Capricorn
>
> **Fixed signs:** Taurus, Leo, Scorpio, and Aquarius
>
> **Mutable signs:** Gemini, Virgo, Sagittarius, and Pisces.

Moon sign: The zodiac sign the Moon was in when you were born. The Moon moves quickly and changes zodiac signs about every 2.5 days. In medical astrology, the Moon represents your energy flow and nourishment needs.

Natal: Referring to the natal or birth chart. The planets' unique locations at the time of your birth are your natal planets. When you see *natal* in front of a planet (i.e., natal Mars), this is referring to Mars in your birth chart and which zodiac sign it's placed in.

Planet: Sun, Moon, Mercury, Venus, Mars, Jupiter, Saturn, Uranus, Neptune, Pluto. In medical astrology, the planets represent body functions or forces that act upon or within the body.

Planetary ruler/ruling planet: Each zodiac sign is ruled by a planet. This planet gives the zodiac sign its primary characteristics. To understand more about a sign, read about its planetary ruler and vice versa.

> **The Sun rules Leo.**
>
> **The Moon rules Cancer.**
>
> **Mercury rules Gemini and Virgo.**
>
> **Venus rules Taurus and Libra.**
>
> **Mars rules Aries and Scorpio.**
>
> **Jupiter rules Sagittarius and Pisces.**
>
> **Saturn rules Capricorn and Aquarius.**
>
> **Uranus shares rulership of Aquarius with Saturn.**
>
> **Neptune shares rulership of Pisces with Jupiter.**
>
> **Pluto shares rulership of Scorpio with Mars.**

Qualities: The four qualities are hot, cold, wet, and dry. All elements, zodiac signs, and planets are made up of these qualities. In medical astrology, the qualities tell us about a planet or sign's physical makeup and what therapeutics are similar or opposite.

Retrograde: When a planet appears to be moving backward from our viewpoint here on Earth. Retrograde cycles are normal, predictable parts of the astrological year and aren't meant to be feared. However, in medical astrology, a retrograde planet may be more likely to correlate with a health condition or healing opportunity.

Rising sign: Also called Ascendant sign or simply the Ascendant. This was the zodiac sign rising up over the horizon when you were born. The rising sign changes multiple times per day and requires an accurate birth time. In medical astrology, the rising sign represents your physical body. When looking at transits to your rising sign, use the exact rising degree.

Station: The pause in motion before a planet changes direction. A planet may station retrograde (backward) or station direct (forward).

Stellium: A group of planets (usually three or more) very close together, or conjunct, in a chart.

Sun sign: The zodiac sign the Sun was in when you were born. When people say, "I'm a Gemini," what they mean is the Sun was in Gemini when they were born. The Sun changes zodiac signs monthly. In medical astrology, the Sun represents your life force.

Transit: Referring to current planetary motion. After you were born, the planets kept moving. This motion and how it interacts with your birth chart are what astrologers call transits. This is an important label because it distinguishes your natal planets from transiting planets, or planets in the sky today. Transits may coincide with significant personal and physical changes. In medical astrology, they tend to present new nutritional, movement, or self-care needs.

Zodiac signs: Aries, Taurus, Gemini, Cancer, Leo, Virgo, Libra, Scorpio, Sagittarius, Capricorn, Aquarius, Pisces. In medical astrology, the zodiac signs represent body parts.

As discussed in chapter 2, in Western tropical astrology, the zodiac signs don't correspond with constellations. They are Earth-Sun relationships. Zodiac signs are 30-degree divisions of the ecliptic, or the apparent annual path of the Sun. This division begins with 0 degrees Aries at the March equinox.

Movement and Fitness Terms

For movement demos from this book, head to
clairegallagher.co/bodyastro.

Agonist/Antagonist: Muscle pairs located on opposite sides of a limb, such as the biceps and triceps or the quadriceps and hamstrings. One acts as a prime mover, while the other is passive.

Bilateral: An exercise that uses both limbs equally, such as a squat.

Circuit: A group of exercises performed in succession with minimal rest.

Conditioning: Exercise that develops the efficiency of the body's energy systems. Although conditioning is cardiovascular in nature, it is not to be confused with long periods of monotonous cardio exercise.

Contralateral: An exercise that uses the arm and leg on opposite sides of the body. For example, a plank where you lift the left arm and right leg.

HIIT: High-intensity interval training. Short bursts of high-intensity exercise followed by short recovery periods.

Intensity: A measure of difficulty, relative to your fitness level. Although there is some crossover, the intensity of aerobic exercise is often defined by how high your heart rate is, while in strength training, intensity is often defined by load (heaviness) and volume.

Ipsilateral: An exercise that uses the arm and leg on the same side of the body. For example, lunging forward with your right leg while simultaneously pressing a dumbbell overhead with your right arm.

NEAT: Nonexercise activity thermogenesis. Refers to energy expenditure that's not intentional exercise. For example, walking to your car, cooking, taking the stairs, and concentrating all use energy.

Plyometrics: Explosive movement that creates power by rapid stretching and lengthening of the muscles. These exercises usually involve jumping.

Tempo: How quickly each portion of a movement is performed. For example, in a squat, there's a downward motion and an upward motion. Taking five seconds to come into the bottom of your squat and then exploding back to the top is an example of a tempo squat. Tempos promote muscle growth by increasing time under tension, or how long a muscle is under strain during a set.

Tempo run: A run performed at an intensity equal to lactate threshold (when blood lactate levels greatly surpass resting levels). This is often called the aerobic/anaerobic threshold. Most of us can't measure our blood lactate, so perhaps a better description is right at race pace, or around 85 percent of your maximum heart rate. When done correctly, this type of training increases your body's running efficiency and threshold over time.

Unilateral: An exercise that isolates one limb at a time, like a single-arm bicep curl.

Bibliography

Bloch, Douglas, and Demetra George. *Astrology for Yourself: A Workbook for Personal Transformation*. Berwick, ME: Ibis Press, 2006.

Casey, Caroline W. *Making the Gods Work for You: The Astrological Language of the Psyche*. New York: Harmony Books, 1998.

Christianson, Alan. *The Adrenal Reset Diet: Strategically Cycle Carbs and Proteins to Lose Weight, Balance Hormones, and Move from Stressed to Thriving*. New York: Harmony Books, 2015.

Cornell, Howard Leslie. *Encyclopedia of Medical Astrology*. Vol. 1. Whitefish, MT: Kessinger Publishing, 2010.

———. *Encyclopedia of Medical Astrology*. Vol. 2. Whitefish, MT: Kessinger Publishing, 2010.

Gagné, Steve. *Food Energetics: The Spiritual, Emotional, and Nutritional Power of What We Eat*. Rochester, VT: Healing Arts Press, 2008.

Gehrz, Andrea L. *Astrological Remediation: A Guide for the Modern Practitioner*. Portland, OR: Moira Press, 2012.

Greenbaum, Dorian Gieseler. *Temperament: Astrology's Forgotten Key*. Bournemouth, UK: Wessex Astrology, 2005.

Hill, Judith A. *The Astrological Body Types: Face, Form, and Expression*. Portland, OR: Stellium Press, 2011.

———. *Medical Astrology: A Guide to Planetary Pathology*. Portland, OR: Stellium Press, 2005.

Hyman, Mark. *Food: What the Heck Should I Eat? The No-Nonsense Guide to Achieving Optimal Weight and Lifelong Health*. New York: Little, Brown, 2018.

Jansky, Robert Carl. *Astrology, Nutrition & Health*. Atglen, PA: Whitford Press, 1977.

Kastner, Joerg. *Chinese Nutrition Therapy: Dietetics in Traditional Chinese Medicine (TCM)*. Stuttgart: Thieme, 2009.

Lehman, J. Lee. *Traditional Medical Astrology: Medical Astrology from Celestial Omens to 1930 CE*. Atglen, PA: Schiffer Publishing, 2011.

Lilly, William. *Christian Astrology*. London, 1647. PDF accessed on sky-script.co.uk.

Lipski, Elizabeth. *Digestive Wellness: Strengthen the Immune System and Prevent Disease through Healthy Digestion*. New York: McGraw-Hill, 2012.

Lynch, Ben. *Dirty Genes: A Breakthrough Program to Treat the Root Cause of Illness and Optimize Your Health*. New York: HarperOne, 2018.

Nauman, Eileen. *The American Book of Nutrition & Medical Astrology*. San Diego: Astro Computing Services, 1983.

Parnell, Deva. *Discovery Yoga Teacher's Manual*. St. Augustine, FL: Discovery Yoga, 2009.

Pitchford, Paul. *Healing with Whole Foods: Asian Traditions and Modern Nutrition*. Berkeley, CA: North Atlantic Books, 2009.

Pursell, JJ. *The Herbal Apothecary: 100 Medicinal Herbs and How to Use Them*. Portland, OR: Timber Press, 2016.

Ridder-Patrick, Jane. *A Handbook of Medical Astrology*. Edinburgh: CrabApple Press, 2006.

Sasportas, Howard. *The Twelve Houses: Exploring the Houses of the Horoscope*. London: Flare Publications; London School of Astrology, 2007.

Thornton, Penny. *The Zodiac Cooks: Recipes from the Celestial Kitchen of Life*. Birmingham, UK: GB Publishing, 2017.

Tobyn, Graeme. *Culpeper's Medicine: A Practice of Western Holistic Medicine*. London: Singing Dragon, 2013.

Tompkins, Sue. *Aspects in Astrology: A Guide to Understanding Planetary Relationships in the Horoscope*. Rochester, VT: Destiny Books, 2002.

Tribole, Evelyn, and Elyse Resch. *Intuitive Eating: A Revolutionary Anti-Diet Approach*. 4th ed. New York: St. Martin's Essentials, 2020.

Index

index

About the Author

Claire Gallagher, MAc, MScN, CSCS, is a post-wellness ally, anti-diet nutritionist, intuitive movement counselor, and medical astrologer. She holds master's degrees in acupuncture and nutrition and is a certified strength and conditioning specialist. Claire uses astrology as a tool for deepening personal authority, self-compassion, and body trust. She's a Virgo Sun, Aquarius Moon, and Sagittarius rising. You can find Claire online at clairegallagher.co.

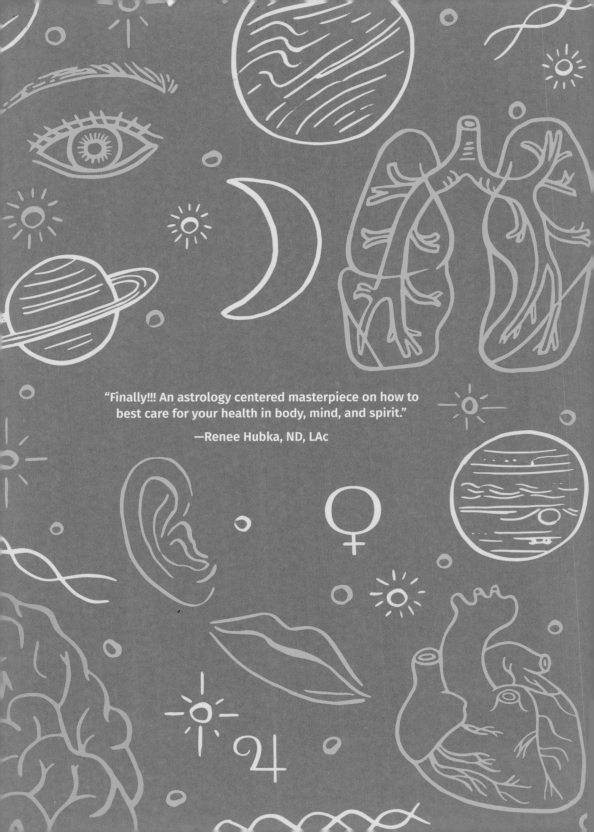

"Finally!!! An astrology centered masterpiece on how to best care for your health in body, mind, and spirit."

—Renee Hubka, ND, LAc